HOW TO BE AN EVEN
BETTER LISTENER

of related interest

Spirituality in Hospice Care
How Staff and Volunteers Can Support
the Dying and Their Families
Edited by Andrew Goodhead and Nigel Hartley
Foreword by the Rt Revd Dr Barry Morgan
ISBN 978 1 78592 102 5
eISBN 978 1 78450 368 0

Chaplaincy in Hospice and Palliative Care
Edited by Karen Murphy and Bob Whorton
Foreword by Baroness Finlay of Llandaff
ISBN 978 1 78592 068 4
eISBN 978 1 78450 329 1

Art of Living, Art of Dying
Spiritual Care for a Good Death
Carlo Leget
Foreword by George Fitchett
ISBN 978 1 78592 211 4
eISBN 978 1 78450 491 5

**Counselling and Psychotherapy
with Older People in Care**
A Support Guide
Felicity Chapman
ISBN 978 1 78592 396 8
eISBN 978 1 78450 751 0

Counselling Skills for Becoming a Wiser Practitioner
Tools, Techniques and Reflections for
Building Practice Wisdom
Tony Evans
ISBN 978 1 84905 607 6
eISBN 978 1 78450 143 3

The Art of Helping Others
Being Around, Being There, Being Wise
Heather Smith and Mark K. Smith
ISBN 978 1 84310 638 8
eISBN 978 1 84642 793 0

Spiritual Care at the End of Life:
The Chaplain as a "Hopeful Presence"
Steve Nolan
ISBN 978 1 84905 199 6
eISBN 978 0 85700 513 7

HOW TO BE AN EVEN BETTER LISTENER

A PRACTICAL GUIDE FOR HOSPICE AND PALLIATIVE CARE VOLUNTEERS

ROBERT MUNDLE

Foreword by **Stephen Claxton-Oldfield**
Afterword by **Greg Schneider**

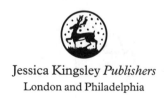

Jessica Kingsley *Publishers*
London and Philadelphia

First published in 2019
by Jessica Kingsley Publishers
73 Collier Street
London N1 9BE, UK
and
400 Market Street, Suite 400
Philadelphia, PA 19106, USA

www.jkp.com

Library of Congress Cataloging in Publication Data
A CIP catalog record for this book is available from the Library of Congress

British Library Cataloguing in Publication Data
A CIP catalogue record for this book is available from the British Library

ISBN 978 1 78592 454 5
eISBN 978 1 78450 829 6

Printed and bound in the United States

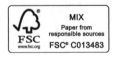

In memory of my father, James Gordon Mundle

This book is dedicated to my wife, Mi-Sook,
and our son, Christopher

Listen to the story told by the reed
of being separated.

"Since I was cut from the reedbed,
I have made this crying sound.

Anyone apart from someone he loves
understands what I say.

Anyone pulled from a source
longs to go back.

At any gathering I am there,
mingling in the laughing and grieving.

A friend to each, but few
will hear the secrets hidden
within the notes."

Rumi, "The Reed Flute's Song"
Translated by Coleman Barks

CONTENTS

FOREWORD

In my role as a university professor, I have been studying and publishing about hospice palliative care volunteers for 13 years. Like others before me, I realized very quickly that volunteers are the heart and soul of the hospice palliative care team. Hospice palliative care volunteers are compassionate and caring people who give freely of their time, energy, talents, and love to support dying persons and their important ones through what is often a terribly difficult time.

In my research, I have spoken with hospice palliative care volunteers as well as coordinators or managers of hospice palliative care volunteer programs. One of the questions I asked was "What makes a good volunteer?" The number-one answer I got from both volunteers and coordinators was "to be a good listener." Here is one anonymous response I was given to the above question that nicely captures the essence of being a hospice palliative care volunteer: "The drive or need to make a difference, a gentle heart, a listening ear, basic kindness, a healthy attitude of death and dying, and an understanding of what the patient and family are facing." It goes without saying that a volunteer is going to be more supportive if he or she is able to offer a listening ear and can also be comfortable with silence—in other words, can "just be" with a patient.

It is absolutely essential that volunteers who are going to be working directly with dying persons and their families receive training to prepare them for their role. One of the training topics volunteers receive is a module on methods of communication and communications skills, with a focus on developing or refreshing active listening, and reflecting on one's communication style. New volunteers want to help, but they often say things like "I wouldn't know what to say to a patient" or "What do we talk about?" *How to Be an Even Better Listener* gives the reader great tips on, for example, initiating a conversation with a new patient. Take a look around the patient's room, and you'll likely find lots of things to talk about, such as personal objects. You can use them to start a conversation and engage patients in their stories. By doing so, you create an opening to be able to listen. Knowing how to listen includes listening with your ears and your body. This book describes how our body language (e.g. amount and level of eye contact) lets patients know that we are interested in hearing what they have to say, and also talks about the importance of "hearing" the feelings behind what a person is saying.

The results of volunteer training surveys show that of all the modules covered in a typical volunteer training program, communication skills are regarded as the most important. It is also the topic that volunteers say they want to know more about. This book provides the "more" about this important topic. Good communication requires more than just talking. It requires good listening as well and throughout the book, Robert offers valuable advice, tips, and strategies in the art of becoming an "even better listener."

How to Be an Even Better Listener is an accessible and enjoyable read filled with wonderful stories told by both dying persons and volunteers. In addition to giving valuable tips on how to listen well, this book also discusses some of the benefits of listening for both patients and volunteers, some of the risks and challenges of listening to others' stories, how telling our own stories benefits us, and how feeling heard and understood not only makes us feel less alone but also makes us better listeners ourselves.

Hospice palliative care volunteers occupy a unique role, often spending more time at the bedside of dying persons than other members of the professional caregiving team. Volunteers consider communication to be the most important topic in their training and have a desire to learn more about it. I agree that it is all about the communication and, in my opinion, *How to Be an Even Better Listener* should be essential reading for all hospice palliative care volunteers as well as healthcare professionals.

Stephen Claxton-Oldfield, PhD, CT
Associate Professor, Mount Allison University

ACKNOWLEDGEMENTS

I gratefully acknowledge the help and support I received from many others while writing this book. The staff and volunteers at Hospice Kingston encouraged my research study, and I thank especially the volunteers who participated in the interviews with me. I thank Ingrid Waisgluss for her lovely translations of the poems "Mas Alla" by German Pardo Garcia, and "La Gran Plegaria" by Alfonso Cortés; Ellie Barton for her thoughtful substantive editing; Natalie Watson at Jessica Kingsley Publishers for her encouragement and support for me to pursue this project; Stephen Claxton-Oldfield for writing the Foreword, and Greg Schneider for writing the Afterword; Sandra Carlton, Neil Elford, and my community of practice at Providence Care Hospital, including librarians Karen Gagnon and Michelle Kennedy. Special thanks to my friend Amanda Quantz, who was a terrific conversation partner for me as we both worked on our separate book projects simultaneously.. Lastly, it is with much love and appreciation that I thank my wife, Mi-Sook, and our son, Christopher, for allowing me the time to devote to my writing. In return, I dedicate this book to them.

PREFACE

In the United Kingdom, there are approximately 125,000 volunteers working in more than 200 hospices (HospiceUK 2017). In France, there are 350 associations of palliative care volunteers with an estimated 6000 members (Tibi-Lévy and Bungener 2017). And in the United States, there are about 500,000 trained volunteers supporting the work of almost 6000 hospices and the patients and families they serve. Of these volunteers, 60 percent assist with direct patient care; 20 percent provide support for clinical care; and 20 percent provide general program support (eHospiceUSA 2016).

What exactly do hospice palliative care volunteers do? According to the French National Palliative Care Association, the tool par excellence of volunteers is *listening* (Tibi-Lévy and Bungener 2017, p.78). And according to one palliative care service in a teaching hospital in Canada, volunteers listen first and foremost; listening is central to their role providing assistance, companionship, and practical support to terminally ill patients and their loved ones (O'Brien and Wallace 2009, p.200). Volunteers have the time to listen. As O'Brien and Wallace put it, "Mostly they bring the gift of time—volunteers take the time to make a difference in someone's day" (p.201).

Some listeners are better than others. Really good listeners are life-giving listeners for those who are ill or suffering in any way, whether it may be physically, emotionally, socially, or spiritually. And they are crucial for those who are struggling to come to grips with the end of life in hospice palliative care.

According to a recent study about the importance of communication skills in end-of-life care (Brighton *et al.* 2017), a majority of participants drawn from hospice palliative care volunteers expressed the need for more training with regard to listening. Participants said that they appreciated especially the training they had received from chaplains, who offered an approach to listening care that helped patients feel valued and heard. These findings echo those of a previous study (Worthington 2008) in which volunteers learned about the qualities of nonverbal communication from a chaplain.

Both of these studies caught my interest because I am a palliative care chaplain and listening is central to my role. Like many chaplains, I see myself as kind of a professional listener (Mowat *et al.* 2013). I am also a clinical educator on topics of spirituality, and grief and bereavement. Over the years, I have had the pleasure of speaking to many groups of hospice palliative care volunteers as part of various training and continuing education programs.

Listening is something we can all learn to do better. As psychotherapist Julia Samuel says, "The ability to listen well is by no means the sole preserve of professional therapists" (2018, p.xiv). If you are a hospice palliative care volunteer, or if you are a healthcare provider who might be wondering why and how to listen better to your patients and their loved ones, then I invite you to continue reading. I help healthcare professionals and volunteers improve their communication skills, and I am ready to share with you what I believe can help you in the art of becoming a better listener.

Robert Mundle

Kingston, Easter 2018

INTRODUCTION

Are you a good listener? I think most people would probably answer "yes" to this question. In my own experience, however, really good listeners are hard to find. In fact, having someone's full attention is so rare to some people that when researcher Caroline Webb (2016) demonstrated to a group of business executives what she calls "extreme listening," which is an approach she borrowed from educationalist Nancy Kline (1999), they told her that the way she was listening to them felt as if she was flirting with them. *Flirting!* Other than flirting, they had no comparable experience of having someone truly listen to them and take such an interest in what they had to say. Similarly, Canadian novelist Robertson Davies imagined that the effect of listening may even seem "hypnotic to someone who has never been listened to, has never had anybody's whole attention, perhaps ever before" (1994, p.213).

I wonder if you can recall a particular time in your life when you were in the company of a good listener, someone who let you speak and who listened to you patiently with their full attention for as long as you needed to talk. Maybe this listener was your mother or father, or a grandparent when you were a child, a close friend, a teacher, or perhaps a counselor, psychotherapist, or spiritual director. Take a moment to reflect on that special experience. What did your listener do or say to show you that she or he was really listening to you? How did that kind of listening make you feel?

I imagine that you might have felt understood, validated, affirmed, valued, relieved, connected emotionally, or even honored to have someone listen to you so deeply. Perhaps the attentive listening you received allowed you to think out loud about a particular challenge you were facing at the time, and helped you to think more clearly and decisively about it—all by being able to express yourself and feel heard. What a gift! That is the real power of listening.

Writer Margaret Wheatley pondered what it is about feeling heard that is so healing for people. "I don't know the full answer to that question," she said, "but I know it has something to do with the fact that listening creates relationship, and we know from science that nothing in the universe exists as an isolated or independent entity" (2002, p.89). In a similar way, drawing upon an article by writer Brenda Ueland (1941), psychiatrist Karl Menninger described listening as "a magnetic and strange thing, a creative force... The friends who listen to us are the ones we move toward, and when we are listened to, it creates us, makes us unfold and expand" (1942, pp.275–276).

Once you have received good listening yourself, you can then recall and draw upon your experiences intentionally to help create those positive feelings in others. Let me give you a few examples from my own life to explain more about what I mean.

I first learned about listening from my parents. As a child, my mother would ask me questions when I got home from school. She wanted to know everything about my day. "What happened next?" she would ask—"You left the house this morning, went down the driveway, turned the corner, *and then...?*" And then I would tell her all my stories, as she continued to ask me for more details. Recalling this memory of how my mother listened to me by asking open-ended questions helps me listen to my patients today in my role as a chaplain in palliative care.

I remember how one of my patients, whom I will call Larry, was telling me stories from his life. In the middle of our conversation, a nurse tried to interrupt us. She was ready to do her morning care with Larry, but Larry wasn't ready for her. He turned towards her and said very graciously, "Excuse me, nurse, I'm trying to tell my life story to this gentleman here, and he's letting me tell it—*the long way.*"

Sometimes it is more difficult to get your listener's attention. At home, my father had an unusual habit of sitting at the kitchen table and eating with his eyes closed. We never knew for sure if he was paying attention to us and our dinnertime conversation or not. In this way, I learned from my father about the importance of eye contact and other forms of nonverbal communication that let others know for sure that you are listening to them.

This reminds me of the children's book *Guess How Much I Love You* by Sam McBratney (1994). I used to enjoy reading it to my son, Christopher, when he was little. I understood well that part in the book where the main character, Little Nutbrown Hare, had to grab his father's long ears when he was speaking to him, "to make sure he was listening."

In my early twenties, I really needed my dad to listen to me. He had come with me on a road trip to Vermont to help me with a business deal I was working on at the time. I appreciated having him with me, because he was so good at providing practical advice. However, as I said, listening was not one of my dad's gifts.

Breaking the silence as we drove, I asked him, "Can I tell you something?" I was at a particularly low point in my life and needed to talk. I wanted to share with him how and why I was feeling so down. His response stunned me. "No," he answered flatly; "I can't handle it." Maybe I should have grabbed him by the ears like Little Nutbrown Hare did to his father, but my dad didn't have a whole lot of emotional capacity for listening. So, we just drove on in a confusing and painful silence. Unfortunately, my experience with my dad is likely typical of how many fathers and sons fail to connect emotionally by not talking and listening to each other.

My point is that different experiences—good and bad—of having other people listen to me have inspired and shaped my way of listening to others in my role as a hospital chaplain. First, I learned how to ask open-ended questions and then to wait patiently for the answers to unfold in stories. Second, I learned how to use body language and nonverbal communication, such as making appropriate eye contact. And third, I worked on developing my emotional capacity for listening, and continue to do so. Finally, I am still learning how to attend to my own needs for self-care, especially when I feel that listening to sad stories is starting to weigh me down.

As part of my formal training I completed a year-long residency in Clinical Pastoral Education (CPE) at the Hospital of St. Raphael, now part of Yale–New Haven Hospital. CPE is a model for learning that combines the action of providing care for those who are ill with reflection on key moments of care. Reflection takes place in a supportive group of peers, and focuses on case reports that describe conversations with patients and family members. I learned how to write case reports as a way to remember meaningful conversations, and to discuss them with others to help identify significant phrases, emotional content, and turning points, as well as any blocks to my listening.

In this book, I want to share with you what I have learned about listening from my personal life and from my professional learning and experience as a hospital chaplain. I also want to share what I have learned by listening to hospice palliative care volunteers like you. I recently completed a research project in which I interviewed individual volunteers about their formative experiences of having someone really listen to them. I have included their fascinating answers in this book to help you in your own self-reflection and learning.

I will present for you key aspects of theory and practice in a variety of stories that are easy to understand. At the heart of all this, I want to explore with you a spirituality of listening— one that is more about the human spirit in general than about religious beliefs in particular.

A lovely spirituality of listening, oftentimes misattributed to poet ee cummings, goes like this:

> We do not believe in ourselves until someone reveals that deep inside us something is valuable, worth listening to, worthy of our trust, sacred to our touch. Once we believe in ourselves we can risk curiosity, wonder, spontaneous delight, or any experience that reveals the human spirit. (McMahon and Campbell 1969, pp.9–12)

If it is true that listening is so significant, isn't it curious that it is so often portrayed in such passive terms as "just" listening, as if it were not nearly as important or effective as "doing" something to "fix" a problem? Skilled listeners, however, know just how active—not passive—listening really is. They know how big a difference there is between being still and doing nothing. They know how challenging it is emotionally and spiritually to "just sit there" and "just" listen, to maintain a "stillness of spirit," and say as little as possible while paying close attention to another person. Listening is *hard work*. In a quotation attributed to theologian and humanitarian Jean Vanier, founder of L'Arche:

> Listening is a difficult and sometimes tedious art. It is so much easier to tell people what to do. But to capture their desires, with an open and free heart, requires a real conversion, a "metanoia," a change of attitude. To listen to someone means to become open and vulnerable to him/her and to allow them to disturb us, to change our habits and our ways of thinking and seeing things. (Quoted in Chang 2006, p.469)

Paradoxically, effective listeners are often most valued and helpful when they are not trying to "do" or "fix" anything at all.

A spirituality of listening requires attunement to subtle gestures and the nuances of "presence." The French twentieth-century philosopher Gabriel Marcel (1889–1973) talked about emotional "presence" in terms of spiritual *disponibilité*. He was referring to a particular kind of emotional and spiritual "availability" in personal relationships.

"The person who is at my disposal," Marcel said, "is the one who is capable of being with me with the whole of himself when I am in need; while the one who is not at my disposal seems merely to offer me a temporary loan—for the one I am a presence; for the other I am an object." And "presence," he said, "reveals itself immediately and unmistakably in a look, a smile, an intonation or a hand shake" (2011, first published 1944, p.42).

Marcel's notion of spiritual *disponibilité* resonates with what Dame Cicely Saunders (1918–2005), founder of the hospice movement, said about the creative spirit of hospice care. Near the end of her own life, she put it this way:

The search for meaning, for something on which to trust, may be expressed in many ways, direct and indirect, in metaphor or in silence, in gesture or in symbol or, perhaps most of all, in healing relationships and in a new experience of creativity. (Saunders 2006, p.275, first published 2004)

Moreover, she said, "those who work in palliative care may have to realize that they too are being challenged to face this dimension for themselves" (p.275). She continued:

Many, both helper and patient, live in a secularized society and have no religious language. Some will, of course, be in touch with their religious roots and find a familiar practice, liturgy or sacrament to help their need. Others, however, will not, and insensitive suggestions in this field will be unwelcome. However, if we can come together not only in our professional capacity, but in our common, vulnerable humanity, there may be no need of words on our part, only of respect and *concerned listening*. For those who do not wish to share their deepest concerns, care is given in a way that can reach the most hidden places. Feelings of fear and guilt may seem inconsolable but many of us have sensed that an inner journey has taken place and that a person nearing the end of their life has found peace. Important relationships may be developed or reconciled and a new sense of self developed. (p.275; emphasis added)

This is the creative spiritual journey I invite you to embark on with me here in this book.

In the chapters that follow, we will take a look at a variety of cues that patients drop for listeners to pick up on and respond to; we will consider three creative approaches to listening, and we will review some helpful things to say in conversations with patients and their loved ones. We will also examine some of the benefits and risks of volunteering in hospice palliative care. And we will raise important questions to encourage you to delve into your own stories to deepen your self-awareness and understanding. I will share with you some of the stories I have collected from hospice palliative care volunteers like you, and offer suggestions about how we can learn from their moving experiences of feeling heard, or longing to feel heard, by significant people in their lives. You will see that each chapter begins with a related quotation from one of the volunteers I interviewed. Finally, I will share with you some details from my own story and my connection to listeners in my life.

Let's continue by taking a closer look at some of the different kinds of heart-rending spiritual needs expressed by patients in hospice palliative care. Then let's explore how we can respond to those needs with more confidence and become better listeners.

You have the time and compassion to listen in your important role as a hospice palliative care volunteer. *Come with me.*

Chapter 1

RESPONDING TO CUES

*We all have different traits, but if you can't listen
you can't be a palliative care volunteer.*
                                        —Ellen, hospice volunteer

In a hospital corridor, a young woman in a wheelchair grabbed my arm. "I don't want to miss something important," she said to me in an urgent voice. She was terminally ill with a brain tumor. "Since I've been sick," she said to me, sobbing, "I've lost my job, I've lost my house, I've lost my friends—I know that I'm dying, and *I don't want to miss something important!*"

By grabbing my arm, I believe she was expressing her need to come to grips with the losses and grief her impending death was imposing on her. *Literally.* She needed to talk to someone before it was too late—someone who would really listen to her, to help her sort out all of her thoughts and feelings, and to help make sure that nothing important was missed. On that particular day, that listener happened to be me. I was in the right place at the right time, and I was available emotionally and spiritually to listen.

How do your patients get your attention when they need to talk? How do they express their need for a listener? I imagine that sometimes their cues might be as obvious as grabbing you by the arm, just as the young woman grabbed me—just like the storyteller compelled his guest to stop and hear his tale in Samuel Taylor Coleridge's "Rime of the Ancient Mariner," with the grip of his hand and "glittering eye" (1997, first published 1884).

Cues might be much subtler too. And there is a good chance, I would even guess, that the signals might be so subtle that sometimes they go unnoticed.

In this chapter, I will introduce you to five of my patients and show you how they got my attention as a listener. Each is presented in a vignette drawn from my memories of real conversations with patients in palliative care over the years. I have changed the names of patients to protect their confidentiality, and I have added some of my own questions and reflections for you to ponder. I would be delighted if these encounters remind you of some of your own experiences of attentive listening as a hospice palliative care volunteer.

Strong men *do* cry

Manny had metastatic prostate cancer. Because he had a prognosis of more than three months to live, he was admitted to the long-term palliative care unit where patients often stay up to a year. He understood, however, that he came to the palliative care unit to die, and sooner rather than later. "I came here to die," Manny said, "and I don't know why it's taking so long." Yet he also talked about having "work" left to do before he died, and how there was "no use dying until you're ready."

Manny was a storyteller. "At ninety-two years old, all I am is stories," Manny said to me. As a story listener, I was hooked. I wanted to hear his stories. However, the stories he needed to tell were very painful for me to hear. He told stories about growing up in a poor family during the Great Depression. And he told many heartbreaking stories of loss and grief across his lifespan, including accidental deaths of childhood friends; the death of his first wife during childbirth the day before their first wedding anniversary; his second marriage with multiple miscarriages and stillbirths; the death of his second wife; and, most recently, the death of his one and only adult son. At the heart of his stories lay an abyss of loneliness.

"If there was a pill for loneliness, I'd take it," Manny said.

The most curious thing about listening to Manny tell his life stories was that I was never sure if he was laughing or crying. It was as if he used laughter to disguise his crying and the deeper emotional pain he was suffering. When he shared his stories of grief and sadness, his voice would quiver, his intonation would rise, his eyes would become large and teary, but he rarely ever actually wept. He told me how as a child his father had taught him that "strong men don't cry." Manny said that his father threatened "to come back from the grave with the devil to get him if he ever cried." Nevertheless, Manny admitted, "my eyes get wet quite often."

As I listened to Manny tell his sad stories and share his feelings about such tragic losses, he gradually started to change. From his assertion that "strong men don't cry"—a belief that is unfortunately typical of so many men—Manny softened his position by realizing "but I'm not strong anymore." He was no longer strong enough to maintain his fearful resistance to expressing how he truly felt inside. And that realization opened the way for his tears to flow.

"All I am is stories," Manny said. Was he saying that with his frail body, nearing death, all he had left of his life were the stories he could tell? Was he feeling kind of like a ghost? Or was he telling me something fundamental about human life itself, that all we ever are, really, at whatever age, are the stories we tell about ourselves? That we live our stories through our bodies? In this way, Manny's tears were his story. From both perspectives, Manny reminded me of how storytellers need listeners, and how important listening can be for those facing the end of life. Telling our stories in the hope of gaining some new insights into their meaning and releasing emotions long repressed can indeed be the work yet to do before dying.

Olga's rosary

Maintaining a sense of personal identity is not easy to do in institutional healthcare settings. A few years ago, researchers in the United Kingdom explored the meaning patients attach to their personal belongings when they move into hospice (Kellehear, Pugh, and Atter 2009). Their study about personal bedside objects in a hospice had two main findings. First, it showed how patients wished to recreate some semblance of "home" in their institutional settings. Second, despite a great diversity of objects, most of which were used for distraction or entertainment, almost every patient harbored at least one personally unique object.

This study reminded me of Olga, a patient I came to know well in palliative care. Among the few objects Olga kept at her bedside was one that was most special to her—her rosary. A rosary is a string of prayer beads, and Olga's rosary looked to me like any other rosary I have ever seen. In her eyes, however, it was unique and special, and she often told me its story.

A priest gave that rosary to Olga while they were both interned in a refugee camp in Poland after the Second World War. From his hands to hers, Olga would put it into my hands too every time she picked it up to show it to me. Then Olga would marvel at how it had never once broken in all the time she had had it.

I took this to be a symbol of Olga's strong faith. As an object of religious devotion, the rosary seemed to me to symbolize her faith in God, and her fidelity to the priest and spiritual friend who lived on in her most heartfelt memory. I think it also symbolized for Olga a deep sense of her own self and personhood—her courageous faith in herself—which was incredibly precious to her in the midst of her steadily worsening dementia that had taken away almost everything else she had to remember herself by. All of these meanings for Olga were typical of the significance of personal objects to older people (Rubinstein 1987).

The significance of Olga's rosary reminds me of a story told by a Brazilian priest and pastoral theologian named Leonardo Boff. In his book on sacramental theology, Boff shared the following story about one of his special objects—his cherished family mug:

> There is this aluminum mug of ours, the good old kind that is bright and shiny. The handle is broken, but that gives it the air of an antique. The family's eleven children of all ages drank from it. It has accompanied the family on its many moves: from rural countryside to town, from town to city, from city to metropolis. There were births and deaths. It has shared everything. It has always been there. It is the ongoing mystery of life and its continuity amid differing situations of life and mortal existence. The mug endures, old but still shiny. When I drink from it, I do not drink just water. I drink in freshness, gentleness, familiarity, my family history. (1987, p.9)

Boff's point is that anything can become a sacramental object, from religious objects like Olga's rosary to something as mundane as an old family mug. The mug is a sacrament for Boff because it represents and symbolizes so much more than what it appears to be on the surface.

Now that I think about it, I remember a set of special family cups at my grandmother's cottage that to me and my family were very much like Boff's family mug. They were bright and shiny too, in metallic colors of blue and red. Every summer I would look forward to seeing them again and drinking from one of them, standing at the sink in my grandmother's kitchen, looking out the window on to the porch and down through the trees into the sunlit yard below. I drank in the whole place from those cups, accompanied by the smell of pine trees, the scurry of chipmunks, the sound of the screen door creaking open and snapping shut again, and my grandmother standing nearby, looking at me, smiling.

These simple cups connected me to my grandmother. They were touchstones for me to the time and place of her cottage, whether I was there in person or only in my mind's eye. And they helped me reconnect with myself too, summer after summer, as I grew older.

I could imagine bringing one of those cups into hospice with me at the end of my life. It would hold such an abundance of meaning for me in feelings and memories, just like Olga's rosary did for her. And it would represent my personal family history to me in a way that anyone within my family would recognize instantly, and that anyone from outside my family wouldn't see or understand at all—unless they happened to ask me about it, and I would tell them its story.

The tree of life

The first time I met Mr. Beech he introduced himself to me with a little joke. "I am the tree of life," he said. Mr. Beech, at the age of 88, saw himself as a beech tree.

He repeated his pun to me in subsequent conversations. It was a "throwaway line" that piqued my curiosity and interest. I am always drawn to stories or phrases that repeat. I hear them as a subtle dangling way to get my attention, an invitation that the person can tuck away again safely if I fail to pick up on the cue. Repetitions might indicate something deeper that people feel a need to talk about. So I asked Mr. Beech to tell me more about how he saw himself as a beech tree and "the tree of life."

"Oh, that was just a joke," he said dismissively.

Perhaps he was surprised that I had taken notice. But gradually he began to explain to me what beech trees are like, including how they are characteristically large, full, and strong trees that provide much-needed food, shelter, and protection to many small animals. This seemed to be significant to his life story. Mr. Beech's love and care for his family was a topic that dominated his conversations with me and with other clinicians and volunteers as well. "My philosophy in life is love," he told me, and his eyes would well up with tears whenever he talked about his devotion to his family. "Without family, you've got nothing," he said.

One of his stories revealed a special poignancy. Embedded in his perspective of a life lived fully over 91 years, with much love and devotion to his family, was a story of enduring loss and grief.

When Mr. Beech was just seven years old, his father died. Mr. Beech explained that his father was abruptly and prematurely "cut down in the crash," referring to the stock market crash in 1929. He and his family believed that his father's stress had been brought on by the financial crisis, and that this had surely been the cause of the sudden fatal heart attack that "cut him down."

I was immediately struck by the recurring metaphor. Mr. Beech saw both himself and his father as a "tree of life." The recurring use of a single significant word or phrase can point to deeper truths (Savage 1996, p.79). This appeared to be true for Mr. Beech's self-identity as a father and provider. Deeper still, it revealed the painful loss of his own father at a young age—a pain that Mr. Beech had been carrying around for most of his 88 years. In Mr. Beech's story, there was intense pain at the roots of his "tree of life," some of which came to the surface in his conversations with me, his listener.

The last of the McLean kids

Listening to Agnes was like trying to follow a newscast on the radio while someone else was slowly changing the channels back and forth across the dial. Agnes had melanoma with metastases to her brain, which caused her to have varying degrees of word-finding difficulties. Jagged words and phrases would erupt in sudden moments of clarity, and then her speech would recede into a garbled backdrop.

Who was Agnes? What was she trying to say?

"I'm the last of the McLean kids," Agnes said to me, crying. I was struck by how her narrative identity of herself as a child was so at odds with her current physical age and appearance. Agnes was 87 years old, mostly bed-bound, and a patient in palliative care who, it seemed to the team, was waiting to die.

According to her physician, Agnes was frustrated with the slow pace of her gradual decline over many months and wished to die as soon as possible. All she wanted was to be reunited with her husband in heaven, he said.

But there was more to Agnes, of course. She was well educated, and she was religious. Psalm 23 was her favorite scripture passage. She spoke in rich symbols and metaphors. And she urgently wanted to tell me something critical about the disturbing dream she had had the night before.

In her dream she was floating down a peaceful river. Carried along by its gentle current, she saw far off in the distance a large door. "Knock and it shall be opened unto you," she said to me. A river is an archetypal symbol, and one that dying patients are known to talk about from time to time (Stanworth 2004, p.19). And the quotation, "Knock and it shall be opened unto you," is from the Gospel of Matthew in the New Testament, where Jesus says, "Ask, and it will be given you; search, and you will find; knock, and the door will be opened for you" (Matthew 7.7, New Revised Standard Version).

While floating down the river towards the large door, Agnes then noticed many obstacles, such as rocks and logs, blocking her way. She explained this by saying, "I get in the way of myself, sometimes." Then she described how she felt that her own will for her life conflicted sometimes with God's will for her life. Later, with great intensity, she said that she had been thinking more about the river and that she wanted to "swim for shore"— that she was looking for a shallow spot along the shoreline where she could stop and rest awhile.

"I'm getting in the river with you," I said.

I took this to be an opportunity to invite Agnes to look back with me over her life and to talk about some of its most important themes, both the flowing water and some of those rocks and logs in her way.

As we floated in the river together, Agnes told me about how she first met her husband 65 years ago, and about the pain of losing him recently. She was lonely.

"At 87 you don't know many people your own age," she explained. "All my friends are gone."

She also talked about her childhood, how she was the youngest child among many siblings in her family of origin, the McLeans, and how she was now the last one living, the last to die—the last of the McLean kids who had been known so well as part of a close-knit family in her small hometown when she was growing up.

The next time I saw Agnes, I asked her, "Are we still in the river?"

"No, the river is gone," she said in a satisfied sort of way. Her urgency was gone.

I took this to be a sign that Agnes was at peace, that her path was now clear. She died shortly after that conversation.

I checked back with Agnes's physician to share with him what I had learned about her. He replied, "Well, patients do say different things to different members of the team, don't they?" Yes, they do. And that's why it's so important to have different kinds of members on a hospice palliative care team, such as physicians, nurses, social workers, chaplains, and volunteers who can take the time to tune in and really listen.

Where the flame departed from the wood

Maria was an elderly Spanish-speaking lady who arrived in the palliative care unit alone and afraid. Her son was far away in another city, and it was difficult for me and other members of the team to get to know her and her needs more fully. Even for the Spanish-speaking physiotherapist on our team, communication with Maria was extremely difficult.

Maria was in spiritual distress, and it was distressing for us to sit with her as she cried out for help. After she settled in a little bit, we learned from her family that she loved to write poetry. We provided her with paper and pens, and then we waited to see what she might write. But there were no poems, or anything else. As we continued to wait, I began to wonder if we had misunderstood the cue from her family.

And then, abruptly, Maria's poetry began to tumble out of her. She began to write out dozens of poems, each on colorful paper in her carefully precise handwriting, one after another. She even gave me two poems as a gift, "Mas Alla" (Beyond) and "La Gran Plegaria" (Great Prayer). I arranged to have them translated into English. Then I framed the originals, and I treasure them to this day.

Màs Allà

Más allá del Silencio, la Armonía.
Más allá de las Formas, la Presencia.
Más allá de la Vida, la Existencia.
Más allá de los Gozos, la Alegría.

Más allá de la Fuerza, la Energía.
Más allá de lo Puro, la inocencia.
Más allá de la Luz, la Transparencia.

Más allá de la Muerte la Agonía.

Más allá, más allá, siempre adelante.
Más allá, en lo Absoluto, en lo Distante,
donde la llama se apartó del leño

a fulgir, por sí misma, en la figura
de un Infinito, va sin Amargura.
Y más allá de lo Infinito, el Sueño.

Beyond

Beyond Silence, Harmony.
Beyond Forms, Presence.
Beyond Life, Existence.
Beyond Pleasure, Happiness.

Beyond Force, Energy.
Beyond Purity, Innocence.
Beyond Light, Transparency.
Beyond Death, Agony.

Beyond, beyond, always forth.
Beyond, in the absolute, in what is distant,
where the flame departed from the wood

O, to glow, by itself, in the figure
of an infinite, now, without bitterness.
And beyond the infinite, the Dream.

(Translation by Ingrid Waisgluss)

La Gran Plegaria

El tiempo es hambre y el espacio es frio
Orad, orad, que solo la plegaria
Puede saciar las ansias del vacio.

El sueno es una roca solitaria
En donde el aguila del alma anida:
Sonad, sonad, entre la vida diaria.

Great Prayer

Time is hunger, and space is cold
Pray, pray, for only prayer
can fill the anxiety of the void.

Dreaming is a solitary rock
where the eagle of the soul nests:
Dream, dream, in everyday life.

(Translation by Ingrid Waisgluss)

Both poems, "Mas Alla" and "La Gran Plegaria," are rich in metaphors and symbols, and they express a deep spirituality and mysticism. At first, I thought Maria composed them. Later, in an internet search, I learned that these poems were written by two Latin American poets, "Mas Alla" by German Pardo Garcia (Columbia 1902–Mexico 1991), and "La Gran Plegaria" by Alfonso Cortés (Nicaragua 1893–1969). I even found a translation of "La Gran Plegaria" by Thomas Merton, the famous Trappist monk, writer, and a poet himself (Tapscott 1996, p.117). Maria had written these poems from memory.

Maria's relationship to poetry raised many questions for me. How did she come to memorize these poems and others? What was her motivation to internalize them, and carry them with her as companions through life? What role did poetry play in her cultural upbringing and identity? What did she wish to express to me through them at the end of her life?

It is possible that Maria had first memorized these poems when she was a schoolgirl growing up in Nicaragua. Recently, I have learned how important poetry is for Nicaraguans. Translator and editor Jessie Sandoval put it this way:

Like most Nicaraguans from my generation, I was raised to venerate poetry, especially that of our Nicaraguan poets... You speak with any Nicaraguan, and they will probably inform you that we are all poets and that Nicaragua is the land of poets—poetry is our most prized export. (2017, p.251)

Maria expressed herself through extraordinary poems that had become part of her very self, in her living, and in her dying. In this way, at the end of her life in palliative care, Maria was able to share with me something deeply important to her about her spirituality and culture.

In addition to what deeper meanings poems and stories might hold for patients, medical sociologist Arthur Frank (2010) suggested that it is also helpful to consider what stories do—how they hail or call us into relationships. Through poetry, Maria called me into a very special healing relationship that bridged language worlds and engaged me on a spiritual level.

Similarly, Patrick Clary (2010), a palliative care physician in New England, said that poetry and metaphors can connect us to the seriously ill, and that such connection can be central to healing at the end of life in a holistic approach to care.

Out of her fear and isolation, Maria connected with me through poetry. I was then able to communicate to the team more about who Maria was as a person. This kind of connection raised her from anonymity to reveal to us one of the most extraordinary patients we ever cared for. Without listening to her through her poetry, I would suggest, we might never have really known Maria at all.

Each of these patients expressed desperate needs for listeners and for listening. They each expressed themselves in stories told through their bodies, and cultures across their lifespans, in their living, and in their dying. There was the strong man who cried,

Olga and her rosary, the tree of life, the last of the McLean kids, and Maria's evocative mystical poetry where the flame departed from the wood.

What each of these storytellers required was a listener—someone to engage them in their stories first of all by picking up on their cues. We saw how these cues can be subtle or overt, and how they were expressed in various ways—in gesture, pun, repetition, personal object, and poetry. These were all cues that signaled something important to notice, pay attention to, ask about, and explore. Cues call us into our roles as listeners. As Janet Dunphy put it, "Listening well, picking up and responding to cues, is an art" (2011, p.26).

Sometimes, however, responding to cues feels too risky. It might take too much of our time, or engage our own emotions too deeply. As Rachel Stanworth (2004) said, the "risk of encounter" explains why caregivers gloss over or ignore cues, like the "throwaway lines" we heard in this chapter—"All I am is stories," "I'm the tree of life," and "I'm the last of the McLean kids." In her observational research at a hospice in the United Kingdom, Stanworth observed how a busy nurse, "without even a sympathetic smile," chose not to respond to her patient's throwaway line that expressed some black humor. Instead, the nurse "simply continued to dress her patient's heels while he explained they were sore because he was kicking the bucket for too long" (2004, p.20).

The important thing to keep in mind is that cues express the *need* for listening. Through cues, patients express a desire to tell their stories. As Arthur Frank explained, "For those who suffer, storytelling is a way out of isolation and way into alliances" (2017, p.5). Storytelling engages listeners. It generates community by turning loneliness into affiliation. In other words, he said, "Stories humanize because they can communalize what has been far too private" (p.5).

Here is one more vignette that illustrates what Frank is talking about and provides another cue to what patients like mine and yours are longing for. It comes from a nursing home resident and is included in a book by Ram Dass and Paul Gorman called *How Can I Help?*

> If they only understood how important it is that we be heard! I can take being in a nursing home. But most people here… they just want to tell their story. That's what they have to give, don't you see? And it's a precious thing to them. It's their life they want to give. You'd think people would understand what it means to us…to give our lives in a story. So we listen to each other. Most of what goes on here is people listening to each other's stories. People who work here consider that to be…filling time. If they only knew. If they'd just take a minute to listen! (2003, pp.112–113)

Understanding well the tremendous need for listeners and listening in healthcare environments, a professor of gerontology at St. Thomas University in Canada by the name of William Randall put it this way: "Narrative care is core care, it's a fundamental element in attending to another person's needs. And it ought to run through everything we do within the health care field—especially where older adults are involved" (2012, p.178).

REFLECTION

- How do your patients get your attention as a listener?

- What are some of the memorable stories you have heard your patients tell?

- Are there any special personal objects that you cherish and keep close by?

  - What awe and wonder do they evoke in you?

  - What relationships from the past do they call forth into being for you now?

- What is your "I am" story or "throwaway" line?

  - I am...

Chapter 2

THREE APPROACHES
TO LISTENING

You have to listen with your ears and with your heart too.
It's like looking at the person with compassion. Gesture,
touch, posture, showing interest are all important.
It's about having your heart attuned to others with
compassion and love that makes the connection.

—Susan, hospice volunteer

In the previous chapter, we explored in a variety of stories some of the cues for listening that hospice palliative care patients expressed. In response to these kinds of cues, let's now explore more about what listening is like in actual practice. As Dr. Danielle Ofri described in her book *What Patients Say, What Doctors Hear*, "listening is one of the most intricate skills we possess, yet also one that seems so obvious we hardly ever think about it" (2017, p.108). So, let's think about it. What does really good listening look like? What does it sound like?

Researcher and listening expert Madelyn Burley-Allen said that listening is one of the "finest strokes" one person can give another person (1995, p.3). In this sense a "stroke" is a form of recognition or attention, like a physical touch, or a nonverbal behavior such as a look, wink, smile, gesture, or the act of listening itself. For Burley-Allen, listening is:

(a) taking in information from speakers, other people or ourselves, while remaining nonjudgmental and empathetic; (b) acknowledging the talker in a way that invites the communication to continue; and (c) providing limited, but encouraging, input to the talker's response, carrying the person's idea one step forward. (p.26)

Building on this definition and appreciation for listening, I would like to offer three approaches to listening to show you how listening to patients can be like reading a novel closely, dancing with a partner, and improvising in a jazz performance. Along the way we will spend some time considering practical recommendations to enhance nonverbal communication, including being at the same eye level, making appropriate eye contact, and maintaining stillness. We will also review some tips to enhance *paraverbal* communication—namely, voice tone, volume, and pace.

Listening is like reading a novel closely

Meet Rita Charon—physician, literary scholar, and founder and executive director of the Program in Narrative Medicine at Columbia University in New York City. Reminiscent of Gabriel Marcel's (2011) understanding of "presence" as spiritual *disponibilité*, Charon described her style of listening to patients in terms of "donating the self toward the meaning-making of the other." For her, listening is a "dramatic, daring, and transformative move," and a "pivotal skill for anyone who wants to be a healer" (2005, p.263). Compared with how listening is so often expressed in passive terms of "just" listening, Charon's appreciation for the power of listening is striking.

In her most recent book, Charon compared attentive listening in healthcare to reading a novel closely. "Close reading," she said, "develops the capacity for attentive listening" (2017, p.166), including "attention to metaphor and figural language, to tone, to mood" (p.169). Close readers take in all the important details. Charon's inspiration is American author Henry James (1843–1916), the subject of her PhD dissertation. Quoting from James's "The Art of Fiction" (1984, p.390, first published 1888), Charon's motto is "Try to be one of those people on whom nothing is lost."

Describing "close reading" in her medical practice, Charon says that she shifts from listening like a doctor to listening like a reader. "My self shifts within my body and consciousness," she said.

> I roll my chair away from the computer. I let my hands sit in my lap. Instead of being on an edge of ignorance and challenge, I feel summoned by the patient—Is it her account? Is it her words? Is it her presence? Is it her action in having come to me because she thinks maybe something good will come of it?—to what feels like a different self, my readerly self. I think it is the difference between being a judging outsider who is being tested to know what to do about a problem, and being a welcoming stranger of its mystery, willing to sit within all its doubts. (2017, p.167)

"This sequence in the office is not unlike a sequence of close reading," Charon explained. "The same alert, creative presence is needed by the reader or the listener; the same attention to all features of the narrating are awakened; the same intimacy between creator and receiver of the narrative is achieved" (2017, p.167).

Hospital chaplains have been applying "close reading" in their own clinical practices for decades. In his book *The Exploration of the Inner World* (1936), Anton Boisen (1876–1965), one of the founders of modern hospital chaplaincy, described his aim to read the patient before him as a "living human document." His approach embodies person-centered care. As he put it, "I have sought to begin not with the ready-made formulations contained in books, but with the living human documents and with actual social conditions in all their complexity" (p.185).

Inspired by Rita Charon's renewed focus on listening in healthcare relationships, I undertook a series of interviews a few years ago with individual hospital chaplains to learn more about how they listen (Mundle and Smith 2013). As a chaplain myself, I know that listening is central to providing spiritual care, but I wanted to hear more from my colleagues about how they listen, and what listening means to them.

The main theme that emerged from these interviews is how important listening is to the role of chaplains in healthcare. All of the chaplains told me stories about how they used listening skills in their daily work, and how they understand listening to be one of the most useful means of caring for people. For example, one chaplain explained how one of his patients called him in his role as a listener to be like a mirror, a recorder, or a kind of container to receive all of her sorrows, all of her pains. In this way, listeners in healthcare environments "hold space" for others in distress.

Another chaplain described listening as paying close attention not only to words spoken, but to *how* they are spoken. Chaplains and hospice volunteers tend to notice important details such as gestures, facial expressions, body language, touch, and tone of voice. They pay attention to these things in other people and in themselves. This is important because, as psychologist Kenneth Gergen mused, "Neurology can tell us much about a blink of the eye, but nothing about a wink" (2009, p.120).

And, as a listening "reader" of people, one chaplain explained to me, "I read emotions in people in how they act and these emotions help me listen better... I take one look at the person and am drawn to them."

Listening to others as "living human documents" is like reading a novel closely. It is also a kind of choreography. Just as Rita Charon described her shift from listening like a doctor to listening like a reader by first rolling her chair away from her computer and placing her hands on her lap to express openness and receptivity to her patients, chaplains and hospice palliative care volunteers also use body language to be better listeners, which leads me to interpret listening as a dance.

Listening is like dancing with a partner

The chaplains I interviewed in my study regarded the following four qualities to be most important to listening and listening well: eye level, eye contact, engaging with emotions as stories, and stillness. I will say a bit more about each of these in turn.

Sit down at eye level with patients

All of the chaplains I interviewed spoke about how their ability to listen well was so often conveyed through their eyes. They spoke at length about how important it is to be at a similar eye level to the person they were listening to. To do this, the chaplains would often need to sit down with patients and loved ones. "The very first thing that comes to mind for listening well," one chaplain said, "is that I sit down. I'm very aware that not many other staff members sit down, and patients and their loved ones really do notice who sits down with them."

Similarly, another chaplain commented:

> I take time with people. I always sit down with somebody when I listen and a lot of the medical staff don't have time to sit down... I find that being at the same eye level with the other person makes listening better, because it tells the other person you're there for them, *and will stay.*

Research has shown that patients commonly perceive that care providers have spent more time at their bedside when care providers sit rather than stand. This is the case even when the actual time spent at the bedside does not change significantly between standing and sitting. Moreover, simply sitting instead of standing at a patient's bedside can have a significant impact on patient satisfaction (Swayden *et al.* 2012).

Let me give you a couple of examples. Having your blood drawn is a fairly routine procedure, but it is also one that is quite invasive. It matters how it is done. This is how two physicians learned to draw blood by sitting down with their patients.

Dr. Kandula is an associate professor at Northwestern University's Feinberg School of Medicine in Chicago. In a video for the American Medical Association posted on YouTube (Kandula 2013), she recalled an interaction with one of her patients who was refusing to have his blood drawn.

"As the intern on the team, it was my job to draw the patient's blood every single day and to monitor his drug levels," Dr. Kandula explained. But when her patient refused to allow her to take his blood, she says that she got "really frustrated and angry" with him. "I started to think about why this is happening, why won't he let me draw his blood?" Then she described the following scene:

> I started to notice that every time I walked into the room he would actually pull out a chair, as if he wanted me to sit down, and I never took the time to do that initially. But one day I actually sat down in the chair, and had an interpreter with me, and actually spent some time asking him if he understood why he was in the hospital, why we were drawing his blood, and why he didn't want me to draw his blood.

It turns out that the patient was afraid of having his blood drawn. Due to a cultural misunderstanding, he thought that it would make him even sicker. Once Dr. Kandula finally understood her patient's perspective by responding to his cue to sit down and take the time to listen to him, she said that "he calmed down a lot, I calmed down a lot, and we were able to develop an understanding. Things were much smoother after that."

At first, Dr. Kandula asserted her authoritative power by ignoring her patient's cues and refusing to come down to his level. *Literally.* Her patient responded negatively by asserting his own power, his autonomy, to refuse treatment. The solution to this impasse depended on Dr. Kandula's willingness to give up some of her authoritative power and accept her patient's invitation to sit down with him, take the time to listen to him, acknowledge his importance as a person, and learn from him what he was thinking and feeling.

The way that Dr. Victoria Sweet learned how to draw blood would be her first experience of what she calls "slow medicine" (2017, p.48). As a medical student, she learned from an expert lab technician how to sit down with a patient.

Whenever I had to draw blood, I would sit down on the patient's bed and make myself comfortable. I would look at the patient, and sometimes we would even smile at each other. It would take more time but I never forgot to take off the tourniquet, and I rarely missed a vein... I had learned that I could sit on the patient's bed, and that sitting created an intimacy, a sharing, a common goal. That getting comfortable, that composing of myself, made a pool of calmness for me and my patient within the crazy cacophony of the hospital. (p.49)

Like Dr. Kandula and Dr. Sweet, the chaplains explained to me that being at the same eye level with their patients by sitting down with them enhances the ability to connect emotionally, to empathize, and to create a feeling of intimacy. In the words of one chaplain, sitting down communicates to others, "I'm like you, I'm not different." As another chaplain put it, "When I come down to their level, it's me joining them where they are and moving with them and helping them travel through unfamiliar emotional territory."

Eye level is also about power. The chaplains I interviewed perceived that moving from a standing position and looking down at others, to sitting and sharing space with others, reduced significant power imbalances in healthcare environments between themselves and patients when listening.

With these points in mind, one of the first questions I routinely ask my patients is "Can I pull up a chair for a moment?" I suppose it is kind of like asking, "Shall we dance?" Then I wait for permission to enter into my patient's physical and emotional space.

Make eye contact

Intimately connected to eye level, the chaplains I interviewed also described how they listened through eye contact. Eye contact is a subtle yet powerful form of communication. Like being at the same eye level, it too extends an invitation. The chaplains perceived that eye contact enhanced their ability to listen by inviting others to share the stories they need to tell and, in turn, to be witnessed by another.

"I make eye contact to listen well," one chaplain said. "I think that might be an invitation to people to tell the stories they need to tell and be heard." Similarly, another chaplain commented, "I make eye contact, I walk over, and before I even introduce myself the patient is pouring out his or her whole story to me." And another chaplain said, "If you make good eye contact, people will start to tell you all kinds of vital things they need to and that you never imagined."

In this sense, for the chaplains, listening became something more than simply a process of *receiving* a story and paying attention to it. To be a good listener was also about actively *inviting* stories—inviting patients to say what they needed to say. Eye contact embodied this invitation, and the quality of that invitation was one of gentleness and respect. It seemed that the chaplains knew that people needed to tell stories to others, but telling personal stories can be very difficult. What is required is another person who invites stories and waits—who does not suppress, teach, preach, or abruptly change the subject.

Making eye contact with patients also helped the chaplains to listen empathically. As one chaplain said, "Eye contact helps me listen better. It helps me empathize, and think about what is going on in the story the person is telling me." Likewise, another chaplain commented, "I think the fact that I'm not rushed, I think the fact that I'm sitting and making eye contact, all of these things are very, very important because they create an empathic bond, and that's healing."

The chaplains embodied in practice what research in neuroscience has been finding about eye contact. Neuroscientist Kai MacDonald (2009) suggested that eye contact between healthcare providers and patients in clinical encounters is potentially valuable for recognizing the presence of unspoken feelings, such as anxiety or shame. This recognition or interpretation of feelings expressed through eye contact, he added, is "part of the basic empathic skills of any clinician" (2009, p.1). He goes on to explain that research on eye contact has found that "mutual gaze and observation of facial responses of others creates a brief, direct link between two minds and automatically engages us in another person's feeling state through neurobiological circuits that create immediate, reflexive, embodied empathy" (p.7).

In simpler terms, I would say that eye contact connects two people emotionally in the personal space between them by the way they see and mirror each other, in their mutual awareness of "I see you seeing me."

That said, however, when making eye contact and seeking to empathize, it is very important to be sensitive to cultural differences. For some people, eye contact can be intimidating, threatening, and inappropriate. Author and educator Nancy Kline learned about this the hard way.

In her courses on listening and what she calls "Thinking Partnerships," Kline used to tell her students to listen by first of all keeping their eyes on the eyes of the other person, and to not look away even for a second (1999, p.44). She taught her students that eye contact is a "basic indicator" of showing one's attention. Then, in an awkward turn of events, one of her students, an Indigenous woman, stood up in one of her classes and said, "Nancy, eye contact is a sign of disrespect in our culture" (p.46). Now she leaves the matter of eye contact to each student's discretion. As a general guideline, however, Burley-Allen suggested that listeners should try to maintain eye contact for about 60 percent of the time in a conversation (1995, p.144). Does that sound about right to you?

Be attuned to emotions manifested in the body

Another way the chaplains explained to me how they listen is by engaging with the physical manifestation of emotions in patients as they tell their stories. Consider for a moment the following scenario. A young child playing outside falls and hurts her knee. Turning and running into her house, it is not until she is in her mother's arms that she bursts into tears. There is something about feeling safe and listened to that allows the release of emotional pain. In this way, the child's tears tell the story of her pain to her mother, in relationship with her mother as an empathic and comforting listener.

In similar fashion, the chaplains were moved by the physical expression of emotion in their patients. Observing these unspoken emotions brought them into a relationship with patients, and in that relationship the chaplains felt a responsibility to listen attentively. For example, one chaplain said:

> Listening to the body, its emotional signs, its actions, tells me a lot about how the person is feeling, who they are too. Sometimes words aren't needed or they just don't have them to say how they feel, so listening to the body is really important. It makes me a better listener. And listening better is for me about knowing we're doing this together. So listening becomes something we all have a responsibility to do too. A person can't do emotions alone, or at least have

them listened to alone. They need others to listen to their tears. Looking at emotions like this also is valuable because I also look at them to feel how they are responding to care.

Attending to a patient's physical expression of emotions also helped the chaplains in the process of listening to sad or horrible stories—stories that others might fear and not want to listen to. As one chaplain put it:

> People's tears don't scare me, it's like, now, okay, we're getting some place, and I'm here to listen. When a person is sad, they often cry, naturally, and the tears come before their words. You can either cut and run or wait to hear the story that is likely to come along.

By listening not only to what patients said but also to *how* they said it—such as the flow of speech, voice control, volume, and intonation—the chaplains commented that they were able to understand how patients felt and how they might be cared for better.

Likewise, the chaplains were able to make meaning out of the tears that come out of a patient's body through the stories they told, and then stay with the sad, fearful, or horrible story that was likely to follow. As one chaplain said:

> Listening to patients' stories helps me make sense of their emotions, whether that is tears or smiles. I think they see in me a comfort with pain and suffering and an ability to move close to them in that time without being overwhelmed or frightened by the immensity of their emotions.

Lastly, a significant part of listening to patients is being attuned to the emotions of others in the wider context of healthcare's narrative landscape. For example, one chaplain said:

> To walk about, to get a sense of what's happening in the hospital, personally, I think it's not difficult to pick up whether people are anxious, busy, if the place is crowded, or empty, what the tone of voice is like of patients, families, and staff. To listen well in general—I see that as part of my job.

Practice stillness

An additional way the hospital chaplains listened is through an appreciation for stillness, by being and having a still body. For example, one chaplain said:

> Listening is hard, but I've come to find that being still is useful. It really helps listening. It makes me calm and lets me keep my attention on them, makes me stay there rather than rushing way, and tells them that I'm not going anywhere. The calm, I think the calm that being still creates in another is something that patients appreciate. We can be in situations and we can de-escalate a lot of times what's going on, just maybe because we're not afraid, because we can allow it to be.

By being still, the chaplains felt a sense of calm that helped inform and maintain their ability to attend to the stories told through the other's body, to stay with the other as the other, and to be there when time is precious. Their stillness spoke to the patient, saying, "I'm here for you, I will stay with your story, your emotions, rather than rush off, leaving you alone, with no one to listen to your tears, fears, and tales of unknown futures."

As one chaplain said, "It's not just about being there, there is something too about the *way* of being there, without a lot of action. As a chaplain, I am not forcing any movement in any direction; it is more like a still point." Or as another chaplain put it, being physically still is useful because "I feel like I can better encourage, pay attention, witness, and be a companion." Stillness also provides a space in which unspoken questions may well up. Whether patients articulate their questions or not, they may sense a yearning within themselves, a need to open up and ask, "What gives my life meaning and purpose?" or "What do I fear most?"

A chaplain in a previous study explained it like this:

If you look like you're going to sit there and listen and be an active listener, rather than someone who is looking at their watch or fumbling with their keys or trying to figure out what the next page is coming in, people will tell you more than you ever really believed they ever would. (Smith 2005, p.99)

Attention to the nuances of body language, including attentive stillness and the subtleties of action and gesture, reminds me of a study completed a few years ago by Brown *et al.* (2011). They confirmed that actions really do speak louder than words in healing relationships, especially when those providing care wish to establish rapport and trust with their patients. "If language is powerful," they said, "arguably the use of non-verbal signs as a means of indicating trustworthiness is more potent still" (p.290). Even "the slightest of gestures" speaks volumes because physical movements are more concrete than vocalizations, and so patients experience gestures more immediately than language.

Moreover, they claimed that "the power of action, especially when it is seen as going beyond that which might be typically expected, was deemed to be especially effective at building trust" (p.291). A good example of this would be how Dr. Rita Charon intentionally rolls her chair away from her desk to meet her patients face-to-face, with her hands placed on her lap in a welcoming gesture that shows her willingness to listen.

For chaplains and volunteers, helpful gestures might also include leaning in when listening to others to demonstrate interest, holding a hand or placing a hand on a shoulder to express care and concern, or offering a smile or other welcoming facial expression (Mundle 2014). As Burley-Allen summarized, "When we listen with an attentive look, lean forward with interest, or have an open body posture, we nonverbally stroke the talker in a positive way" (1995, p.27). You might do many or even all of these things already in your role as a volunteer.

If nonverbal aspects of listening make listening kind of like dancing with a partner, let's now consider the soundtrack that goes along with it.

Listening is like jazz improvisation

To teach communication skills to their medical students at Penn State Hershey Medical Center, Dr. Paul Haidet and colleagues (2017) use jazz music as a metaphor. In their elective course called Jazz and the Art of Medicine, they draw on the styles of many different jazz musicians to help their students think about and reflect on styles of communicating and how they can become effective listeners to their patients.

The challenge, according to Dr. Haidet, is that many medical students believe that "medicine is characterized by linear, cause-and-effect problems best solved only by algorithmic and deductive thinking" (Haidet *et al.* 2017, p.3). So, instead of providing students with lists of best practices and key phrases to memorize and use in conversations with patients, the instructors invite students to listen to some of the great voices in jazz history and learn from musicians how to improvise and communicate effectively.

The improvisational part of jazz is much like human conversation, the researchers explained (p.2). Through jazz, students come to appreciate the use of silence, pacing, communication latencies (the time between turns at talk, or what I would call "pause time"), and open-ended questions. By comparing and contrasting the styles of various jazz singers and musicians, students learn how to draw out and listen for deeper meanings in patients' stories, and they learn how to develop their own authentic voices as communicators.

In one exercise, students listen to two recordings of the same song, "They Can't Take That Away from Me," composed in 1937 by George and Ira Gershwin. Do you know this song? It was composed for the film *Shall We Dance* starring Fred Astaire as Peter and Ginger Rogers as Linda. Through the lyrics, Peter notes some of the small endearing things he will miss about Linda. "The way you wear your hat, the way you sip your tea," and "the way you hold your knife, the way we danced till three." Each verse is followed by the line, "No, no, they can't take that away from me." The basic meaning of the song is that even if the lovers part or become physically separated, the memories cannot be forced from them. Thus, it is a song of mixed joy and sadness. In Dr. Haidet's class, the medical students might relate the song to how they got to know their patients, and what they might remember fondly about each of them.

The medical students listen to versions of the song performed by Sarah Vaughan (1924–1990) on her album *Swingin' Easy (1957)*, and by Billie Holiday (1915–1959) on her album *Songs for Distingué Lovers* (1957). Both versions were released in the same year, and they are performed in the same key and at the same tempo. Naturally, however, each interpretation of the song is very different. After listening to both versions of the song, the students share their comments about which one of the singers, Sarah Vaughan or Billie Holiday, they would most like to "be like" as a physician.

You can try this exercise for yourself. For me, the choice is clear. As a communicator and listener in palliative care, I would rather be like Billie Holiday in her version of the song. Don't get me wrong, I think Sarah Vaughan and Billie Holiday are both great singers. But I hear Sarah Vaughan's version of "They Can't Take That Away from Me" to be more about her than anyone else. It is youthful-sounding, and fun, but I also hear in it a mocking tone at times. At one point it even comes to an abrupt halt in an awkward-sounding pause. As a recording, and as a metaphor for listening in healthcare, it also lacks for me solos by the accompanying musicians and the opportunity to hear their voices as well.

In contrast, Billie Holiday's version is more subdued and seductive. It is more heartfelt, relaxed, and wise, and it sounds more appreciative of the person she is singing about. The best part for me is that Billie Holiday as a singer invites and draws out long solos from her accompanying musicians. In a word, it sounds to me like a conversation—an intimate, shared, and co-creative musical conversation. In my opinion, it is an excellent metaphor for how a conversation with a patient might unfold in a respectful, artful, and meaningful way. What do you think?

To summarize, listening is an important way to recognize and pay attention to another person. It is a way to provide care by "reading" another person and responding in creative and authentic ways. We have explored how healthcare staff and volunteers might approach listening creatively by drawing upon its similarities to reading a novel closely, dancing with a partner, and improvising in a jazz performance.

Because healthcare is so unpredictable, it is helpful to draw upon approaches to listening that are like spontaneous, thoughtful improvisations in movement and voice. This can be especially helpful in heartfelt encounters between patients and caring listeners who enter together into uncharted territory through storytelling and conversation about what matters most in the end. In these kinds of relationships, listeners are crucial to drawing out and even *co-creating* another person's stories and expression of feelings in close partnership and caring collaboration. As Randall, Prior, and Skarborn explained, listeners are not merely "neutral instruments for gathering objective data." Rather, they help shape stories as "pivotal players" in dynamic processes (2006, p.382).

REFLECTION

- How would you describe your own approach to listening?

- What does it feel like for you to make eye contact?

- Do you notice any differences in the quality of your conversations with patients when you sit and when you stand?

Chapter 3

HELPFUL THINGS TO SAY

When someone really asks you a question and listens, you have the opportunity to be reflective. It makes you wholly present when you are the center of somebody's focus.

—Irene, hospice volunteer

In this chapter, we will take a look at some of the most helpful things you can say, and not say, in your caring conversations with patients and their loved ones.

What those who are suffering need to hear from you

People often struggle with what to say to those who are suffering. They can struggle so much that they end up saying things that sound awkward and strange. You may have felt this way as a volunteer. If you have, that is understandable. It may be reassuring to know that it is okay to admit that you don't know what to say.

"Your words don't have to be wise," Yale theologian Nicholas Wolterstorff said. "The heart that speaks is heard more than the words spoken. And if you can't think of anything at all to say, just say, 'I can't think of anything to say'" (1987, p.34). It is honest, and it frees you from overthinking and maybe even trying too hard to be helpful. Wolterstorff's recommendation comes from his own personal experience of heartbreaking loss.

Following the death of his son, Eric, in a mountain-climbing accident when he was 25 years old, Wolterstorff said:

> What I need to hear from you is that you recognize how painful it is. I need to hear from you that you are with me in my desperation. To comfort me you have to come close. Come sit with me on my mourning bench. (p.34)

Philosopher Havi Carel wrote about her experience of her own life-limiting respiratory illness, diagnosed when she was in her mid-30s. She too expressed what she needed to hear from others. "Several times," she said, "when I told people about my illness they asked: 'So how long do you have?' The question always left me gasping for air" (2008, p.123). Like Wolterstorff, she invited caring listeners to simply be with her in her pain and loss, and to focus more on listening than speaking.

> What I learned from my illness is that in times of hardship, grief and loss, there is no need for original, illuminating phrases. There is nothing to say other than the most banal stuff: "I am sorry for your loss"; "this is so sad." Saying this— and listening—are the best ways to communicate with ill people. (p.58)

When six dying patients were interviewed in a PBS documentary on the end of life, called *On the Edge of Being*, one patient, who was himself a physician, offered the following critique of his colleagues, who were caring for him:

What I expect from you is that you hear my questions. I know that you don't have the answers. I know that I have questions to which nobody has the answer. But struggling with me, with my questions, you show me respect. You value me by listening to my questions. (Quoted in Smith 2005, pp.57–58)

Listening to questions keeps conversations alive and it keeps the focus on the patient. Pat answers, explanations, clichés, or, worst of all, advice that we might be tempted to give, shut down conversations and patients.

Start conversations by requesting permission

Your patients might feel open and ready for a conversation. But maybe not. Opening up questions and talking about feelings requires attention and energy, and the timing needs to be right for patients. It can also be risky for them. Therefore, it is helpful to begin by first asking a basic closed-ended question: "Do you feel like talking?" Or, as I suggested in the previous chapter: "Can I pull up a chair for a moment?" The answer you receive could be a simple "yes" or "no."

Respond to feelings

Sometimes your patients might begin by expressing some strong feelings, such as anger, that appear to be directed at you. If a patient says something like "I'm dying, I feel awful, and you're no help," it can be difficult not to take it personally. But as Dr. Robert Buckman explained, you have some choices at this point. You can react to the judgment "you're no help" by saying defensively, "Well, I'm doing my best." Or you can focus on how the patient is feeling (1988, p.25). A simple but helpful response could be something like "I'm really sorry to hear that." Then you could take your cues from what happens next. The patient might tell you to "Get lost!" Or the patient might offer to you some indication of wanting to talk, either in words, or in a look, or in a reflective silence. As a first step, acknowledging feelings invites dialogue and allows others to say more about how they are feeling, if they wish to do so.

Paraphrase

For psychotherapist and author John Savage, paraphrasing is the first skill listeners need to master. By paraphrasing, you let patients know that you are paying close attention and seeking to understand what they are saying. As Savage explained, "Paraphrasing is the act of saying back to the speaker in your own words what you heard the person say" (1996, p.23). However, he also acknowledged that it is not easy to do.

> At first, you may think that paraphrase skill is easy, and for some it is. But for most of us, it takes a great deal of concentration. It is not possible to paraphrase what others verbally communicated to you if you did not listen to what they were saying. This means that the listener must give full attention to the speaker. (p.23)

Following are some phrases you can use to reflect back in a paraphrase what you heard, or think you heard, and to check with your speaker if you heard her or him correctly.

- You are saying that... Is that correct?

- What I hear you saying is that...

- If I am hearing you right, you are...

- Let me say what I am hearing...

Check your perceptions and interpretations

Taking a further step beyond paraphrasing, a perception check is "checking out your guess at another person's emotional state" (Savage 1996, p.39) if it is not clear already. By sensitively seeking to identify and acknowledge another person's emotions and feelings, you express care and concern. Based in observation, a perception check conveys your attention, and because you express it indirectly as a well-intentioned guess, it is a non-threatening way to invite patients and family members to confirm what they are feeling, and to share more details if they wish to do so.

Here are some examples of how to check your perceptions about how a person might be feeling.

- Is it possible that you might be feeling...?

- I notice that... I wonder if...

- I get the impression that...

Perception checks are a gentle and respectful way to offer to listen to more of a person's story without breaching the need for privacy or raising his or her defenses.

Similar to checking your perceptions, you can also check your interpretations of the deeper meanings embedded in the stories you are hearing, like Mr. Beech's recurring "tree of life" metaphor, in Chapter 1. But first, Savage cautioned, you should ponder your relationship with the speaker. Do you and the patient have a relationship of sufficient rapport and trust that the patient will want to open up to you? If you attempt to explore deeper meanings before you have built trust and rapport, you may be met with resistance and denial. "If you do a check without appropriate rapport," Savage said, "people may consider it an invasion of privacy and become resentful and emotionally distant from you. When you have built strength in the relationship, then the check is perceived as caring and helpful" (1996, pp.98–99).

Similarly, pastoral theologian Pamela Cooper-White cautioned, "One should never impose interpretations or state another's need for him or her" (2004, pp.128–29). Rather, she argued that humility is required (p.129) whereby "the patient is not an 'It' to be acted on, but a 'Thou'" (2007, p.243). The goal, she said rightly, is "to be with the patient not as the expert who will tell him or her who s/he is, but as a respectful guide to his or her own winding journey in the *selva oscura*, the forest full of shadows" (p.243).

Ask open-ended "quality" questions

Take a moment to recall the last time you felt deeply connected with someone in a conversation. "Chances are," Caroline Webb says, "it involved the other person showing some real curiosity about your life and your views" (2016, p.118). And it probably involved what she calls "quality questions"—the kinds of questions that shift the quality of any conversation. Quality questions are *qualitative*, open-ended questions that can't be answered with a simple "yes" or "no." They build rapport by inviting people to share their thoughts and feelings, and their own questions, over merely facts.

Let me give you some examples. Elizabeth Mackinlay is a registered nurse, Anglican priest, and author. In her book *Palliative Care, Ageing and Spirituality* (2012), she suggested that the following open-ended questions are appropriate and helpful to ask people of all different cultures and faiths. By asking these kinds of qualitative questions, volunteers can help draw out patients' thoughts and feelings, and demonstrate not only curiosity and interest, but also concern and care.

- What gives greatest meaning to your life now?
    - What is most important in your life?
    - What keeps you going?
    - Is life worth living?—Why is it worth living? If not—why not? (This question is especially important now in light of medical assistance in dying in Canada.)
- Looking back over your life,
    - What do you remember with joy?
    - What do you remember with sadness?
- What are the hardest things for you now?
- What do you look forward to now? (p.46)

Of course, it also matters *how* you ask these kinds of questions. Qualitative researchers Mills, Speck, and Coleman explained that it is helpful to ask these kinds of questions in a hesitant, accepting, and gentle manner. This encourages people to feel relaxed and less anxious when responding. To ask these kinds of questions in a hesitant manner is a sign of respect that acknowledges the personal and private nature of potential answers, and it honors the emotional struggle, how hard it is to engage these kinds of questions and issues. It also gives others time and space to think about their answers without feeling rushed (2011, p.38). This quiet approach is particularly important when listening to older adults who might struggle with finding the right words to express their beliefs and values, and who might find it embarrassing to try to do so unless the listener is patently interested in their search for meaning (p.57). *Listening takes time.*

Another open-ended question that can be especially helpful and meaningful in hospice palliative care is "What else are you hoping for?" Sometimes patients and their loved ones can get stuck emotionally by hoping for just one thing, such as a miraculous cure to an incurable disease. It is natural for patients and their loved ones to hold on to this kind of concrete hope. How could they not? Yet those who work and volunteer in healthcare might consider this kind of hope to be "false" hope, and it is difficult to know what to say in response to it.

A good example of this kind of conundrum appears in Dr. Paul Kalanithi's moving memoir of his own terminal illness, *When Breath Becomes Air.* He described receiving the horrible news of his diagnosis, followed by his father's desperate attempt to provide emotional support in the form of concrete hope for a cure. Dr. Kalanithi recalled the narrative his father supplied immediately in the face of their fear—"I was going to beat this thing, I would somehow be cured." Dr. Kalanithi reflected, "How often had I heard a patient's family member make similar declarations? I never knew what to say to them then, and I didn't know what to say to my father now." Then he asked himself the following open-ended qualitative question: "What was the alternate story?" (2016, p.127).

Alternate stories could be about hope, and how the things we hope for can change. A true tenet of medicine is not to take hope away (Sweet 2017, p.153). But what if the patient and family seem to be hoping for the wrong thing—the impossible? In this situation, one Catholic physician suggested that they shouldn't lose hope. "Perhaps instead of hoping for a miracle, what they should hope and pray for is that they find the strength to accept what's happening" (Smith 2005, p.47).

In a similar way, hospice chaplain Maria Drews recommended that listeners try to "diversify hope":

> Without directly challenging the hope for a miraculous cure, we can help patients and their families diversify their hopes by taking a "yes, and..." approach. Say "yes" to their hope for a cure, miracle, or long-term survival, but follow up with an "and" statement, adding other hopes the patient and their family have shared. For example, validate their hopes, even false hopes, by saying, "I would like to see that for you, too," then ask, "What else are you hoping for?" (2017, p.14)

Qualitative, open-ended questions invite broad, reflective answers. They take alternative stories into consideration, and these possibilities may lead to more questions. As chaplain Drews put it, "We never stop hoping, we just change what we hope for" (p.14).

Say, "tell me more"

Are you the type of listener who is willing to hear more? Or do you wait impatiently for an opportunity to jump in and start telling your own story? Good listeners don't follow up qualitative questions with their own comments right away, nor do they offer simplistic practical advice to complex emotional problems.

Instead, according to Caroline Webb, "merely by saying 'Tell me more about that', you'll be in the top percentile of listeners that anyone will meet today" (2016, p.119; Ueland 1941). It also helps you as a listener to keep the conversation going. Nodding or saying affirmative things, such "Yes," "I see," or "Tell me more," sounds simplistic, but in stressful situations, Robert Buckman said, "it's the simple things you need to help things along" (1988, p.17).

Expect humor and initiate it when appropriate

Is humor appropriate in palliative hospice care? *Yes!* Research shows that humor is important to patients nearing the end of life and that it arises frequently in hospice visits (Adamle and Ludwick 2005; Claxton-Oldfield and Bhatt 2017). Common types of humor include jokes and riddles, reading a funny story to patients, and even gallows humor that makes light of topics that are usually considered unpleasant, painful, or taboo, like death and dying. In Chapter 1, we heard the pun Mr. Beech repeated about his name, "I'm the tree of life," and we heard the gallows humor of the patient who told his nurse that his heels were sore because he had been "kicking the bucket" for so long.

Humor can help build rapport and ease tension. According to Adamle and Ludwick, "It is an integral supportive measure that creates a safe and comforting environment for patients," and it requires "moment-to-moment listening and unconditional acceptance" (2005, p.289). But as Claxton-Oldfield and Bhatt rightly point out, it requires volunteers to read and take their lead from their patients' cues (2017, p.421).

To summarize, good listening is an active way of providing care by offering your attention to the facts, and, more importantly, the feelings, that someone is seeking to express. Creative listeners provide emotional space for others to reflect more deeply and express more fully their thoughts and feelings by asking permission, responding to feelings, paraphrasing and checking their perceptions and interpretations to make sure that they are truly understanding the other person, asking open-ended "quality" or qualitative questions, offering to hear more details, and being open to hearing whatever their patients might wish to say and talk about, including humor. These are some of the critical skills every listener needs.

REFLECTION

- What are some of the most helpful things others have said to you when you have felt unwell? What are the most unhelpful comments you have received?

- What does it feel like for you to say "I don't know what to say"?

- Have you shared some jokes and humor with your patients? What was that like?

Chapter 4

BENEFITS AND RISKS OF VOLUNTEERING

As a volunteer, I'm driven by need.

—Ann, hospice volunteer

In previous chapters we looked at what listening is like in actual practice. We considered some creative approaches to listening, and we reviewed qualitative open-ended questions and other helpful things to say in conversations with patients and their loved ones.

In this chapter, we will consider some of the potential benefits and risks that listening poses for patients and volunteers alike in hospice palliative care, and we will take a look at some questions that we can ask ourselves to reflect on and assess our own complex needs.

Benefits and risks for patients

Drawing new life from old stories

Family members and friends have likely heard their loved one's stories many times before, and everyone may be stuck in a well-worn groove. As Randall and McKim explained, "contact with the same old interlocutors can mean staying stuck in the same old stories" (2008, p.170).

Alternatively, new relationships with healthcare staff, especially with volunteers, create new opportunities for patients to tell their stories. Arthur Frank (2017) observes that even transitory moments of having someone listen can create feelings of shared experience and community. And new listeners provide more than just fresh ears for old stories. They can ask new questions of storytellers to draw out more details from their stories and to explore potentially new or broader meanings that were perhaps previously overlooked or forgotten.

For gerontologist William Randall, taking time to listen as well as possible creates opportunities for patients to unpack and open up their stories from "cramped versions" they might feel them reduced to in the present (2012, p.187). This kind of attention to narrative potential enhances care for the whole person by helping patients feel more respected, appreciated, and more deeply themselves (Randall 2012; Randall and McKim 2008, pp.117ff.).

Randall quoted theologian and spiritual writer Henri Nouwen (1976) who said, "Healers are hosts who patiently and carefully listen to the story of suffering strangers. Patients are guests who rediscover their selves by telling their story to the one who offers them a place to stay" (Randall 2012, p.187).

Hospice chaplain Kerry Egan is a good host. In her listening care for her patients and their loved ones, she sees herself as a story holder. "We listen to the stories that people believe have shaped their lives," she said. "We listen to the stories people choose to tell, and the meaning they make of those stories" (2016, p.17). Recalling the many stories she has heard in conversations with her patients over the years, she described how her patients benefitted "often, but not always," by finding as they talked "some measure of peace," how their faith was affirmed in something good and greater than themselves, and how they found strength they didn't know they had to make amends with the people in their lives, and courage to move forward without fear of death (p.4).

Along with the potential benefits that listening offers to patients and their loved ones, there are also risks of harm. Risks stem from the raw physical, emotional, and spiritual vulnerability that patients and their loved ones experience as death approaches in palliative hospice care.

Be prepared for different reactions

One risk has to do with initiating new relationships in healthcare situations; it matters how rapport and trust are established and built. In their recent study, Tibi-Lévy and Bungener documented four distinct reactions patients and their loved ones have to hospice palliative care volunteers: they can be positive, distant, mistrustful, and even hostile (2017, p.67).

Consider how you might feel if someone you have never met before starts asking you questions about your personal thoughts and feelings, and about your life history. In return, you might ask the following kinds of questions about her or him. Who is this person? Do I feel comfortable with this person? What roles and responsibilities does she or he have in relationship with me? Is the personal information I share confidential, or will it be shared with others? What difference would that make to me?

When hospice nurse Heather Meyerend enters a patient's home for the first time, she knows that she "is walking into a long, long, complicated story that she understands nothing about, a story that is reaching its final crisis" (MacFarquhar 2016).

Unlike nurses who work in hospitals, Meyerand's approach to care is "purposely inefficient"—she moves slowly; she sits down; she delays; she lingers. When journalist Larissa MacFarquhar spent some time with Meyerend on home care visits, she observed how Meyerend embodies the philosophy of hospice care in how intentionally available she is "to chat, to sit close by, to put her hands on the patient's skin as she goes about her checkup."

> Her visit may be the high point of the day for the patient, who may not be able to get out of bed, or for whoever is taking care of the patient, who may not have left the house or seen anybody else for a day or two; either or both of them may be going a little crazy and may badly need interruption or variety of any kind, ideally someone different to talk to. (2016, p.2)

Unfortunately, patients and their loved ones might not always welcome or appreciate the care and support that staff and volunteers offer. This might come as a surprise to volunteers and other health-care staff who want to be helpful. Like nurses and other healthcare staff, volunteers might find themselves drawn into complexities of family relationships and emotional dynamics, including rivalries and conflicts between family members about unresolved issues. They might encounter patients and family members in their feelings of grief and anxiety, fear and denial about what is happening, and guilt and uncertainty about what they should do and what needs to be done (MacFarquaur 2016). In this swirling mix of intense feelings and emotions, volunteers might find themselves included or excluded in circles of care, trusted or rejected, depending on how patients and their loved ones see them and understand their role.

Stirring up painful memories

Another risk for patients has to do with feelings roused in life review. The unexamined life isn't worth living, Socrates said—to which writer Kurt Vonnegut added, "But what if the examined life turns out to be a clunker?" (quoted in Hitchens 2017, p.70). Sadly, life review doesn't always lead to resolution or peace of mind; it can stir up, disturb, and trouble one's thoughts and feelings.

Drawing upon the work of psychologist Robert Butler (2007), Randall and McKim explained how, depending on the intensity of the conflicts patients are wrestling with, life review can lead to fear, depression, and even suicide. For some, it might lead to the tragic recognition that they haven't truly lived their life at all, that their years have in many ways been wasted. In this respect, "life review can be the route, not to reconciliation but to regret, not to serenity but to despair, not to writing a satisfying ending for one's story but to shutting it down" (2008, p.227).

Hospice nurse Heather Meyerend appreciates that sometimes patients want to talk to her about their life because it is easier to talk to a stranger than with a family member, or because she isn't a therapist, or just because she is there and available to listen. She also respects that some patients don't want to talk about their past. Sometimes there is just too much pain for them to deal with. Holocaust survivors she has nursed, for example, usually don't want to talk about it (MacFarquhar 2016).

Is it worthwhile for patients to share their life stories with you? Only they can say, of course, and only if they know the potential risks and benefits. Sharing their stories might not lead to feelings of peace and closure. Nonetheless, Butler (2007) appreciated how it can lead to greater self-knowledge. That alone, he said, is a virtue in itself (cited in Randall and McKim 2008, p.227). But in some situations, your patients and mine might feel that the potential benefit of greater self-knowledge is too costly.

Finalizing others

An additional risk for patients is what Frank (2004) called "finalization." This has to do with the information listeners hear, or think they hear, and what they do with it next. For example, instead of expanding narrative possibilities and details for patients, it is possible for listeners to "finalize" their patients by summarizing their stories inaccurately and inappropriately, as if their stories somehow expressed their definitive "last word." This can happen when we begin to talk not *with* our patients, but *about* them.

There is always the possibility for listeners to "get it wrong" and for someone to say, "That's not what I said or meant." Just think of the "telephone game," for example, where a message changes as it's repeated down the line from one player to the next. At the end of the line, the original message can be unrecognizable to the person who started it. The game illustrates how quickly messages can be altered as they are relayed from person to person, even in a relatively short timeframe. As a game, it can be funny. In real life, however, it's like gossip. And in healthcare, it's unethical, particularly when we don't check with our patients directly to make sure that we have heard them correctly.

Finalization might come also in the form of listeners identifying too closely with what their patients say. The most common example of this is when someone says, "I know how you feel." No doubt this statement means to express empathy, understanding, and connection between two people. But it comes across as "finalizing" stories by the way it pivots away from the speaker's story and shifts the focus on to the listener's own supposedly related experience.

While it can be appropriate for me to *guess* how you might be feeling, and then to confirm it with you by checking my perceptions as discussed in Chapter 3, it is impossible for me to know *exactly* how you feel. I don't know what it is like to be you, and you don't know what it is like to be me. That is why when someone says to me, "I know how you feel," I hear a harmonica start to play in my head, followed by Tom Petty's voice singing "You Don't Know How it Feels," from his album Wildflowers (Petty 1994).

My point is that there is always more to any person's story. Stories are never *complete* (Kenyon and Randall 1997, p.154); no listener ever hears the whole story and no teller ever tells it (Randall *et al.* 2006). Consequently, good hosts never "finalize" their guests; they remain open to whomever their guest may become (Frank 2004, p.46).

Benefits and risks for volunteers

Mutual healing

Hospice palliative care volunteers, like you, value their role as listeners. Research has shown that the opportunity they have to listen to their patients' life stories is one of the main things that keeps them volunteering (Claxton-Oldfield and Jones 2013). One possible reason is that listening to someone's story creates intimate life-giving connections and empathic bonds in a heightened situation rarely experienced in everyday life. Would you agree?

The experience of listening can even be healing for storytellers and listeners alike. Researchers Boston and Mount concluded from their study about caregivers in palliative care, including volunteers, that "when a meaningful caregiver–patient bond existed, healing occurred not only for the patient but also for the caregiver" (2006, p.25). When hospice chaplain Kerry Egan reflected on how her patients benefitted "often, but not always" from her listening care, she then said about herself, "always, they taught me something" (2016, p.4).

What did she learn?

Egan learned that everyone has a story. "When you talk to hundreds of people who are dying and looking back over their lives," she said, "you come to realize something startling: Every single person out there has a crazy story. Every single person has some bizarre, life-shattering, pull-the-rug-out-from-under-you story in their past" (p.17).

Through listening to other people's stories, Egan learned to accept her own story. "Just as it was true for every one of my patients," she said, "something had happened to me too" (p.5). In this way, she learned that everyone, including herself, is in some way "broken and cracked." And being "broken and cracked" is not necessarily the end of Egan's story or anyone else's. It is not the final word. "I don't know if listening to other people's life stories as they die can make you wise," she said, "but I do know that it can heal your soul. I know this because those stories healed mine" (p.5).

Being broken and cracked, repaired and healed, evokes archetypal images and symbols. The "wounded healer" in Greek mythology, for example, presents a model for Christian ministry (Nouwen 1972), for narrative ethics in healthcare (Frank 2013), and for appreciating the "spirituality of imperfection" in all kinds of healing relationships (e.g. Kurtz and Ketchem 1992). From the iconic Liberty Bell in Philadelphia comes Leonard Cohen's famous poem "Anthem":

> Ring the Bells that still can ring
> Forget your perfect offering
> There is a crack in everything
> That's how the light gets in.

> (Cohen 1993, p.373)

Another good image for this kind of healing from being "broken and cracked" emotionally and spiritually comes in the form of Japanese pottery known as Kintsugi ("golden joinery"). Kintsugi is the Japanese art of repairing broken pottery with lacquer that is dusted or mixed with powdered gold, silver, or platinum. Approaching the story of objects philosophically, it treats breakage and repair as part of their history, something to highlight and appreciate, rather than something to disguise or hide.

Writing about Kintsugi for *The Washington Post*, journalist Blake Gopnik (2009) described an exhibition at the Smithsonian museum called Golden Seams: The Japanese Art of Mending Ceramics. "Because the repairs are done with such immaculate craft, and in precious metal," he said, "it's hard to read them as a record of violence and damage."

> Instead, they take on the look of a deliberate incursion of radically free abstraction into an object that was made according to an utterly different system. It's like a tiny moment of free jazz played during a fugue by Bach.

Strong emotional reactions

Alongside the benefits for hospice volunteers are the risks of strong emotional reactions to illness and suffering, dying and death. Volunteers might experience intense feelings of sadness, grief, anxiety, vicarious traumatization, exhaustion, and eventually even burn-out. Confronting illness to listen attentively to those who are ill is hard work, and it taxes listeners physically, emotionally, and spiritually.

Philosopher Havi Carel observed the emotional impact that her own life-limiting illness had on her visitors. "People feel terror, embarrassment and mortification when they are confronted with illness," she said. "Some respond to these emotions by confronting them, others by fleeing. Some overcome the initial sense of panic and surprise; others run a mile, from me, from illness, from themselves" (2008, p.57).

For Elizabeth Tova Bailey, it was the same thing. In her illness memoir, *The Sound of a Wild Snail Eating*, she described what it was like to be bed-bound for months with a debilitating and paralyzing illness. From her bed, she observed her visitors observing her. "I was a reminder to them of all they feared," she said—"chance, uncertainty, loss, and the sharp edge of mortality." As she put it, "those of us with illnesses are the holders of the silent fears of those with good health" (2010, pp.39–40).

Meeting suffering

Illness evokes anxiety in others, and anxiety inhibits listening. The impulse is to look away, change the channel, change the subject. Yet the crucial ethical challenge for listeners, Frank explained, is "not to steer the storyteller away from her feelings" (2013, p.101). Steering clear of feelings only denies what is being experienced and compounds the loss. Instead, he concluded that what is needed, specifically in clinical work, is "enhanced tolerance," or what I would call emotional *fortitude*, for meeting suffering head on as part of life stories.

Yet Frank's ethical imperative is not met without significant struggle. It is extremely challenging to confront the shock of illness in order to listen attentively and care for the person who is ill. This is true for a patient's close friends and family, for volunteers, and even for professional listeners, such as hospice chaplain Kerry Egan. As she put it,

If you think it's not work to stay steady, to remain present, to not pull back in the face of terrible suffering, then you have never been in the face of terrible suffering. It's something I've failed at. I try not to flinch, I try not to be overwhelmed, I try not to run away. But I have. (2016, p.20)

Seeing others in your patients

Do your patients and their families ever remind you of someone else, such as your own family members, friends, or maybe even yourself? This is called countertransference. Transference affects how your patients see you; countertransference refers to what you see in them—your own feelings, attitudes, or desires, positive or negative, that you attribute unconsciously to the other person in caregiver–patient relationships.

According to Boston and Mount, "The challenge for care providers is to become aware of the aspects of their own suffering that they are projecting onto the patient and to reflectively work with these aspects of the self" (2006, p.19). Listeners risk projecting on to others their own beliefs and values, fears and hopes, desires and aversions. Consequently, they might misrepresent the other's views, needs, and concerns, and arrive at interpretations or moral judgments that are inaccurate and inappropriate (Mackenzie 2006).

Maintaining boundaries

It is important for listeners to respect personal boundaries in therapeutic relationships, particularly the "otherness" of patients—to remember that caregiving relationships are between people who are mutually other. For Frank, "Seeking to enter the other's life seems generous, but it risks losing the mutual otherness that sustains the boundary between persons and thus sustains a fundamental condition for dialogue" (2005, p.295).

So the goal of listening and empathizing is not to internalize the feelings of the other, but what Dr. Jodi Halpern (2001) called "resonance" with the other. To listen well to others is to resonate with their stories, to feel them reverberate or echo within us, without allowing them to settle in or get stuck there. In this way the other's story does not become my own; I can appreciate the story being told and feel its nuances without having its emotional weight overwhelm me.

Listening might not help

While active listening can be helpful, it isn't *always* helpful in *every* situation. For some people, having access to an active empathic listener, who appears to have unlimited amounts of time to give, can create or sustain feelings of dependency. Just as patients and their loved ones can get stuck in the grooves of the same old stories, so too can patients get stuck with healthcare staff and volunteers. The result could be that even while trying to listen actively to a patient, we might not feel very actively involved in the conversation at all. Despite our best intentions and efforts, it might feel that the listening we can provide is not making much of a difference. Instead of helping others, it can drain and exhaust us.

Therefore, it is helpful to be aware of limits for yourself when you sit down to listen to others, including limits on your time and on your ability to help. I know that I can listen attentively for about an hour at a time at the most. It is also helpful to keep in mind that you can refer to other members of the hospice palliative care team when you feel that the needs you are facing are beyond your scope or expertise as a volunteer.

The good news about the risks volunteers and healthcare staff face as care providers is that we can use the thoughts and feelings that are stirred within us to provide better care and support to others; we can use them to learn more about ourselves, our own motivations, limits, and needs.

Reflective assessment

For patients, family members, and caregivers alike, the realm of serious illness can trigger feelings of existential aloneness and disintegration of self (Boston and Mount 2006). In response to the potential for strong emotional reactions to illness, Boston and Mount emphasized the need for caregivers to monitor and assess their own personal emotional cost of being a palliative caregiver, as well as their needs for informal and formal support (2006, p.24).

Let's take a look at some questions that you might include in your own ongoing reflective self-assessment.

What kind of energy do I bring? Do I use it in a helpful, healing way? How do I know this about myself?

Elizabeth Tova Bailey expressed how eagerly she awaited her visitors. Like the golden seams in Kintsugi ceramics, she described how her friends were "golden threads randomly appearing in the monotonous fabric of my days" (2010, p.38). Bailey needed her visitors to be present and available to her—physically, emotionally, and spiritually. She needed her visitors to match the quiet energy of her own attentive stillness. Yet she was astonished by the random way her friends moved around the room. "It was as if they didn't know what to do with their energy," she said, "they were so careless with it" (p.39). Observing her visitors, she noticed how it took time for them to settle down.

> They sat and fidgeted for a while, then slowly relaxed until a calmness finally spread through them. They began to talk about more interesting things. But halfway through a visit, they would notice how little I moved, the stillness of my body, and an odd quietness would come over them. They would worry about wearing me out… Eventually, discomfort moved through my visitors… Their energy would turn into restlessness, propelling their bodies into action with a flinging of the arms or a walk around the room; a body is not meant to be still. Soon my visitors were off. (pp.39–40)

Jill Bolte Taylor described in *My Stroke of Insight* (2008) how at 37 she experienced a rare form of stroke in the left hemisphere of her brain that left her unable to walk, talk, read, write, or recall any part of her life. It took more than eight years of rehabilitation therapy for her to recover. In the midst of her chaos she needed her visitors to bring her positive energy. "It was very difficult for me to cope with people who came in with high anxious energy," she said.

> I needed people to come close and not be afraid of me. I desperately needed their kindness. I needed to be touched— stroke my arm, hold my hand, or gently wipe my face… I really needed people to take responsibility for the kind of energy they brought me. We encouraged everyone to soften their brow, open their heart, and bring me their love. Extremely nervous, anxious or angry people were counter-productive to my healing. (pp.125–126)

The energy that visitors provided Jean-Dominique Bauby was his lifeline. In *The Diving Bell and the Butterfly* (1997) he described how he faced the horror of "locked-in syndrome" following a severe stroke that nearly killed him. Almost completely paralyzed, he could communicate only by blinking his left eyelid. Remarkably, by such tenuous connection to various dedicated listeners, Bauby dictated his thoughts and feelings letter by letter to the outside world.

"It is a simple enough system," he explained, "you read off the alphabet (ESA version, not ABC) until with a blink of my eye I stop you at the letter to be noted." Repeating this maneuver for each of the letters that followed, Bauby was able to spell out whole words, and then fragments of sentences, paragraphs, until, eventually, he completed his book. That was the theory. In practice, however, some visitors fared better than others. He explained,

> Because of nervousness, impatience or obtuseness, performances vary in the handling of the code (which is what we call this method of transcribing my thoughts)… Nervous visitors come most quickly to grief. They reel off the alphabet tonelessly, at top speed, jotting down letters almost at random…they take charge of the whole conversation, providing both questions and answers… Meticulous people never go wrong: they scrupulously note down each letter and never seek to pierce the mystery of a sentence before it is complete. Nor would they dream of finishing a single word for you. (pp.29–30)

How do others experience us as listeners? Does our emotional energy allow us to receive the stories others need to tell? Illness narratives such as Bailey's, Taylor's, and Bauby's help us understand not only what it is like to be seriously ill, but what it is like for patients to receive visitors. They turn the tables on healthy and able-bodied visitors to allow us to see the types of physical energy we bring, and our emotional capacity, or lack of capacity, to be present to those who need us most.

Bauby's story especially reminds me of an encounter I had with a lady in palliative care who was dying from liver cancer with lung metastases. Severely jaundiced, with irregular breaths, she could only whisper one word at a time, with pauses so long between each word that I thought she had fallen asleep. Waiting for her next words to come I sat close beside her. Leaning in to hear her, I found that I too became very still and quiet, and that my energy, my breathing, slowed to match hers. Synchronized with her, I listened as she said, fadingly:

> They...used...to...call...me..."the...miracle...lady"... because...I...beat...cancer...so...many...times...But... not...this...time.

In the brief connection we shared, she was able to give me an encapsulated version of herself, word by word, until it was completed. Her story summarized her relationships, her identity, her relief, her struggles, her letting go. Yet each of these topics was a cue to so many more details that we could have explored more fully together if the circumstances were different.

But maybe the questions she cued for me speak more to my needs than hers. Through listening to her I felt my own need to have someone listen to me too, just as patiently and attentively, to help me piece together my story.

What are my needs?

Sometimes caregivers become so focused on meeting the needs of others that they forget to pay attention to their own needs. Meeting the needs of others might be an unconscious way of meeting our own needs. And caregivers might not even acknowledge that they have needs of their own at all, to receive care themselves. Has this ever happened to you?

In this chapter, we have reviewed some of the benefits, risks, and challenges of listening for both patients and caregivers alike in hospice palliative care. While listening can provide new opportunities for empathic bonds and healing relationships that are mutually beneficial to patients and volunteers, listening is not always helpful in every situation. We also explored some of the risks and challenges raised in listening relationships that can influence how patients and their loved ones welcome and receive volunteers, or not. Volunteers and other caregivers might even distance and exclude themselves from some situations when the emotional struggle to meet suffering head on becomes intolerable. Navigating the impulses and dynamics of finalization, countertransference, and emotional energy calls for deeper self-reflection and assessment facilitated by the questions we raised.

REFLECTION

- What needs of my own am I meeting by volunteering in hospice palliative care?

- What kinds of emotional energy do I carry? How do I know? Have I ever asked for or received feedback from others about how they experience my energy?

- What kinds of patients or situations rouse strong feelings and emotions within me?

- How much sadness and grief am I taking on?

- Do I know my boundaries and limits?

- What kind of support would be most helpful to me?

- How do I care for myself?

- Who is this "self" that I'm supposed to care for? *Who am I? How have I changed?*

Chapter 5

YOUR OWN STORY AND GRIEF JOURNEY

I never have these types of conversations
where people ask me questions that lead me to
delve into my spiritual life or my fears.

—Gary, hospice volunteer

To go deeper, to really listen to the stories of other people, it helps to listen more fully to our own stories as well. As Kenyon and Randall put it, "We need to make our own story available to ourselves as a prerequisite to really being able to listen to another's story" (1997, p.150). The more we know about ourselves, the more available we can be physically, emotionally, and spiritually to listen to others. The more deeply I am able to listen to myself, the more deeply am I able to listen to others. In other words, depths of self-reflection reveal to me possibilities for "deep" conversations with others and give me the freedom to listen to their needs and issues without my own getting in the way.

Yet so many of our experiences go unacknowledged, and the stories we could tell about them remain untold. They are hidden from view, perhaps because they are too painful to talk about. Unfortunately, the result could be that if someone wants to talk to me or to you about something we haven't addressed in our own lives, or at least acknowledged to some degree, we might not be able to ask the right kinds of qualitative questions about it and listen attentively to the stories that follow. We might even change the subject.

"Taboo" subjects like money, sex, politics, and religion are best avoided at family gatherings, aren't they? They make people uncomfortable and trigger arguments. Perhaps the biggest taboo subject of all these days is death. Culturally speaking, death used to be more openly acknowledged. Older adults might remember family members dying at home. And they might remember attending wakes. But these traditions are fading. Funerals are transitioning into "celebrations of life," and grief is abbreviated by unrealistic cultural expectations to "get over it" as quickly as possible.

In this chapter, we will consider how to make our own stories more available to ourselves. We will peer into the dark regions of death and grief to learn from them. Our guide to this kind of self-reflection will be the late-Romantic Austrian composer and conductor, Gustav Mahler (1860–1911). Loss and grief marked Mahler's life all the way through. But what he did with his sorrow is astonishing. Through his creative self-expression he transformed suffering into beauty. Before we get to that, however, let's explore some general questions for self-reflection to open up some of our own stories.

Everyone has a story, and more than just one. There are multiple stories within our stories. Reflecting on our personal narratives is important because it can help us connect more deeply to ourselves, more emotionally to others, and more significantly to the transcendent or what some might call the sacred dimension of life.

Let's begin by considering one of life's biggest questions— "Who am I?" We might begin to answer it by simply stating our age, gender, family role, and saying something about our job or vocation. In this way I would describe myself as a middle-aged husband, father, and hospital chaplain. But there is more to me than that, of course. Much more.

What *kind* of person are you? According to your personality type, you might be introverted or extroverted, or a mix of both. Are you a thinker or more of an emotional person? I imagine that you are someone who likes to help others, but what are your needs, your passions? You might also reflect on whom you love, and who loves you. What seizes your imagination, what gets you out of bed in the morning, what breaks your heart, and what amazes you with joy and gratitude (Arrupe 2009)? There are dozens of topics for self-reflection, and each one can trigger memories and evoke stories that you could tell about yourself.

With my love of music and philosophy, I am inspired by how philosopher Cornel West (2008) described himself by saying, "I'm a bluesman in the life of the mind, a jazz man in the world of ideas." I like how jazz bassist Charles Mingus (1922–1979) struggled to describe himself by saying, "In my music, I'm trying to play the truth of what I am. The reason it's difficult is because I am changing all the time" (Hentoff 2001, p.99). And I like how playwright and psychologist Florida Scott-Maxwell landed a series of cultural counter-punches in her autobiography, written when she was in her eighties. "We who are old," she said, "know that age is more than a disability. It is an intense and varied experience...something to be carried high... My eighties are passionate. I grow more intense as I age" (1968, pp.5, 13–14). I too grow more intense as I age, emotionally and spiritually.

You might jot down a few descriptive phrases about yourself. Perhaps there is one that captures nicely for you the essence of who you are.

Next, you might sketch out some of the key stories you tell repeatedly about yourself. As an example, theologian and humanitarian Jean Vanier summarizes his life in a few brief stories. Vanier is the much beloved founder and beating heart of L'Arche—the non-profit, faith-based organization located in 50 countries worldwide. In L'Arche, people who have intellectual disabilities, and those who come to assist them, share life and daytime activities together in home-like family settings that are integrated into local neighbourhoods. At 90, Vanier continues to live in the original L'Arche community he founded in Trosly-Breuil, France, more than 50 years ago.

In frequent interviews and talks about his life and ministry, Vanier routinely tells three stories about his life that are fundamental to his understanding and appreciation of his personal development and identity. He talks about *trust*, *inspiration*, and *vocation*.

Vanier recalls how at 13 he told his father that he was going to join the Royal Navy. His father's response? "I trust you."

Still in the midst of the war, I told my father that I wanted to cross the U-boat-filled ocean to join the Royal Navy College in blitzed southern England. His answer to me was, "I trust you. If that is what you want to do, you must do it." My father's trust in me confirmed my trust in myself. When he said, "I trust you," he gave me life; he gave me permission to trust my intuitions and to just do what seemed right. I knew that if he trusted me, I could trust myself and others to do what was right. (2007, p.2)

Next, he talks about his inspiration to start L'Arche in the 1960s after he visited a similar small community founded near Paris by Fr. Thomas Philippe, a French Dominican priest. "My first meeting with Père Thomas was deeply moving... Listening to him, simply being with him, I felt transformed and I felt a presence of God" (p.3).

And of his vocation in life, Vanier explains that his "essential vocation" is "to discover who I am and what Jesus wants of me" (Znaimer 1990).

Few of us are as saintly as Jean Vanier, but his focus on trust, inspiration, and vocation in his life prompt us to consider these topics in our own lives. Is there something significant that someone said to you growing up that gave you life, gave you permission to trust yourself, to trust others, and to do what you feel is right? Who would you say in your life history inspired you the most? And what would you say is your "essential vocation"? How did you choose to become a hospice volunteer? What does volunteering mean to you? Answers to these kinds of questions provide focus and direction that can be especially helpful in times of uncertainty.

Pastoral theologian Melissa Kelley invites us to reflect on the following kinds of core questions in order to enhance our approach to helping others. What are the plotlines of our life stories, the major and minor characters, and themes? She asks:

How are past, present and future connected in your story? Is your story sensible and coherent? What parts of your story have you learned and absorbed from your family, from your culture, from your faith tradition? What other sources have shaped your story, for better and/or for worse? (2010, p.93)

Next, she asks about meaning in our life stories:

> What is the meaning embedded in and expressed through your story? How does your story reflect how you understand sense, purpose, and significance in your life? How does your story communicate what you value, what your priorities are in life are, and what you believe? How does your story express how you understand yourself? How does your story reflect how you understand God's feelings about and responses to you? (p.93)

And she addresses loss: "When have you experienced loss, what has happened to your story and your meaning system?" (p.93).

Each loss and each person's experience of grief is unique, and it might be hard to put it into words. Instead, if you were to draw your journey through one particular loss, what would your grief look like? What colors would you use? What shape would it take? Would your drawing depict progression through grief?

Sometimes people draw grief as a journey through a valley. Following the shock of loss, your drawing might show a descent to the bottom. Then it might move forward horizontally until, at some particular point, it begins to ascend up and out of the valley. In this way forward, you might show how your grief moved through different stages, such as denial, anger, bargaining, depression, and acceptance (Kübler-Ross and Kessler 2005).

Alternatively, your grief might look like a chaotic jumble of feelings and emotions that shift abruptly back and forth between experiences of grappling with loss, on the one hand, and ways of setting it aside, on the other—bracketing it—in order to attend temporarily to other pressing matters of daily living (Stroebe and Schut 1999). Your drawing might be a scribble that shows movements back and forth. Whatever form it takes, how you express your grief will reflect your own unique experience.

We expect that grief will be "healing" in a straightforward manner. But that is not always the case. Following the sudden death of her husband, writer Joan Didion reflected on her experiences of grief in light of the split between "grief as we imagine it" and "grief as it is." She presumed that "a certain forward movement" would prevail, and that "the worst days will be the earliest days" (2005, p.188).

> We imagine that the moment to most severely test us will be the funeral, after which this hypothetical healing will take place... We have no way of knowing that the funeral itself will be anodyne, a kind of narcotic regression in which we are wrapped in the care of others and the gravity and meaning of the occasion. Nor can we know ahead of the fact (and here lies the heart of the difference between grief as we imagine it and grief as it is) the unending absence that follows, the void, the very opposite of meaning, the relentless succession of moments during which we will confront the experience of meaninglessness itself. (pp.188–189)

Who would ever expect the intensity of grief to peak at six months, or nine, or even a year after a loss? That we never really "get over it"? Not entirely. So, what do we do with grief? How can we express it creatively, in meaningful ways that are helpful for ourselves and others?

To answer these questions, let's look to the life of composer Gustav Mahler to open up some more topics for self-reflection and discovery.

Mahler

Viennese composer and conductor Gustav Mahler (1860–1911) described himself in a short phrase: "I am thrice homeless," he said, "as a native of Bohemia in Austria, as an Austrian among Germans, and as a Jew throughout all the world" (A. Mahler 1973, p.109). That restlessness fuelled his creativity. He composed massive works of symphonies and symphonic song cycles for voice and orchestra. Today, his music is among the most often performed and recorded of all composers. In universal themes of alienation, death, and grief, but also of hope and joy, Mahler poured his intensely personal emotions into music that stirs the hearts of listeners worldwide.

In his personal life, Mahler shifted abruptly between feelings of joy and sadness. His facial expression would suddenly change "from cheerfulness to gloom," conductor Bruno Walter (1941, p.128) observed.

It seemed as if he were reproaching himself for having thoughtlessly forgotten to remember something that was sad... At the bottom of his soul lay a profound world-sorrow whose rising cold waves would seize him in an icy grip. (p.128)

As his wife Alma recalled, "Mahler seldom felt happy when he went out anywhere. His gloom was infectious. Everyone felt as if 'there was a corpse under the table'" (A. Mahler 1973, p.65). There were *many* corpses, in fact.

Mahler was the second child of 14 in a family marked by multiple deaths. First, there was Isadore, Mahler's elder brother, who died one year before Mahler was born. Thereafter, Mahler witnessed childhood deaths beginning when he was five years old. Five more of Mahler's brothers died in infancy of diphtheria, and a sixth, Mahler's beloved brother Ernst, died at age 12 of hydrocardia after a long illness.

Psychologically speaking, Dr. Stuart Feder explained, "For the child who experiences sibling death repeatedly throughout childhood, its serial meanings range from unawareness to bewilderment and confusion; to the mysterious and magical; to superstition and feelings of guilt; and finally, to anxiety" (2004, pp.60–61).

Mahler responded with music. At age five or six, he wrote his first composition—"Polka with Introductory Funeral March." Out of his experience of death at such a young age, Mahler the satirist was born (p.143).

But that is not all. In 1895 Mahler's beloved brother Otto died by suicide at age 21. He shot himself. According to Alma, "he left a note saying that life no longer pleased him, so he handed back his ticket" (1973, first published 1946, p.9). Mahler's eldest sister, Leopoldine, died of a brain tumor at age 26 in 1899, the same year that Mahler's father and mother both died. And Mahler last saw his brother, Alois, in 1904 at the train station in Vienna where he departed for America. Only two family members, Justine and Emma, remained in Mahler's life.

Yet there is more. In 1907, when he was only 47, Mahler was diagnosed with a fatal heart disease. "That I must die is no news to me," he wrote to Bruno Walter.

But without attempting here to describe or to explain that for which there are perhaps no words at all, I merely want to say that, at one fell stroke, I have lost everything of clearness and assurance that I had ever won for myself; and that now, at the end of my life, I must learn anew how to walk and stand. (Walter 1941, pp.150–151)

Sadly, there is even more. The same year that Mahler was diagnosed with heart disease, his first child, Maria (nicknamed "Putzi," meaning "little one" or "cute one"), died at age four of scarlet fever and diphtheria. Alma's marital infidelity three years later, in 1910, was only the most recent loss in a life-long trail of loss and grief. One year later, at 50, Mahler was dead.

Conductor Bernard Haitink (1996) put it this way, "Mahler was a man who suffered and who had a talent for suffering, his whole life was a fight against everything...and you hear that in his music." He mourned through music. He poured his grief into art songs, such as in the *Rückert Lieder*, especially the haunting song, "Ich bin der Welt abhanden gekommen" (I Am Lost to the World) (1901); the song cycle *Kindertotenlieder* (Songs on the Death of Children) (1904); and the last movement, "Farewell," of Das Lied von der Erde (The Song of the Earth) (1909).

Theodore Reik (1983), one of Freud's first students, heard in Mahler's setting of poems by Friedrich Rückert (1788–1866) memory traces of grief and sorrow for two of Mahler's siblings in particular—Isadore, who preceded him, and Ernst, one year younger than him, who died in 1874. Did Mahler feel "survivor guilt" over his deceased brothers? Mahler mourned his brothers in *Kindertotenlieder* as well, especially Ernst whom he knew, loved, and cared for. Pain and loss mark every one of its measures.

Reik described how, in *Das Lied von der Erde*, Mahler "filled those songs with all the grief and anxiety he experienced... The summer of 1908 was full of grief. Stirred to the depth by the death of his child and worried about his own bad health, Mahler could not be diverted. The only thing in which he found peace of mind and satisfaction was work on the *Lied von der Erde* and on his *Ninth Symphony*" (1983, p.350). In the fluttering motif in the first movement of the *Ninth Symphony*, some listeners, following conductor Leonard Bernstein, hear the sound of Mahler's ominously irregular heartbeat.

Mahler sought not only to express his feelings of grief through music, but to transfigure death into life. Powerful examples of this occur in the *Second Symphony*, subtitled "Resurrection," the *Fourth Symphony*, in which the "Dance of Death" is transformed into angelic "Heavenly Life," and the finale of the *Ninth Symphony*, in which death music is transfigured into a hymn to life.

The third movement, "Ruhevoll" ("quiet," "peaceful," "restful"), of Mahler's *Fourth Symphony* opens with the cellos playing a gentle cantilena, a lyrical instrumental melody (Mahler 1966). I can't think of a more serenely beautiful piece of music, especially in the recording of Otto Klemperer (1961) conducting the Philharmonia Orchestra. The theme is stated and then varied, melodically paraphrased, extended, and combined with a distinctive counter-melody in the violins and later in the oboe (Floros 2000, p.127). The musical dialogue builds to a tender climax in the highest register of the violins, shimmering quietly above the cellos as they cycle slowly downward, punctuated by pizzicatos in the basses and harp. It sounds to me like the separation of the heavenly life from the earthly life. Without losing sight of each other, however, the cellos turn back, take a small step upward, and reach out to the violins at the very moment the violins swoon. It is one of the most heartbreakingly beautiful melodies I have heard.

To borrow a phrase from literary critic George Steiner, this moment "mends my heart in the breaking" (1989, p.97). Or, as neurologist and music lover Oliver Sacks said, "Music can pierce the heart directly; it needs no mediation... While such music makes one experience pain and grief more intensely, it brings solace and consolation at the same time" (2007, pp.329–330).

Feeling, thinking, breathing, suffering—music represented for Mahler the whole human being (Floros 2000, p.12). As Walter explained, "His sorrow and his yearning became music, and just as they were reborn again and again, so they were turned ever anew into a work of art" (1941, p.131).

Mahler and Freud

Mahler's *First Symphony* is ambitiously heroic, known as "The Titan." His *Second Symphony* is even more monumental. It is scored for large orchestra, two vocalists, and chorus. "My whole life is contained in my two symphonies," Mahler said. "In them I have set down my experience and suffering, truth and poetry in words. To anyone who knows how to listen, my whole life will become clear" (quoted in Feder 2004, p.7).

Yet near the end of his short life, his pain unbearable, Mahler sought connection with a different kind of listener. Instead of symphony patrons in public concert halls, not all of whom understood or appreciated his music, Mahler poured out his heart in a private meeting with a psychoanalyst—none other than Sigmund Freud.

In the summer of 1910 Mahler sent a telegram to Freud, requesting a consultation. By that time both men were prominent figures in Vienna and practically legends in their respective fields of music and psychoanalysis. Just as Mahler knew of Freud's reputation in the emerging field of psychoanalysis, Freud knew also of Mahler's reputation as an accomplished conductor and prolific composer.

Freud was on holiday with his family in Leiden, Holland. "I made an exception by receiving someone during my vacation," Freud said, "but a man like Mahler!" (quoted in Feder 2004, p.209). From Tyrol, Austria, Mahler travelled the nearly one thousand kilometers by train to Leiden to meet Freud. During their meeting they strolled around the town for four hours while Mahler divulged his pain in words and conversation.

According to Feder, "Mahler customarily used such walks in the company of intimates to work through personal conflict as well as creative problems" (2007, p.212). Before he met his wife, Alma Schindler, it was Natalie Bauer-Lechner who filled this role. While Mahler talked, expressed, and vented, Natalie walked quietly at his side, "questioning, eliciting, but above all, listening" (p.212).

Walking around the university town of Leiden on that Friday afternoon in August 1910, Mahler and Freud would have looked like two academic colleagues engrossed in conversation. As Feder imagined, "Freud, with his walking stick and student's stoop might have appeared to be one of the professors" (p.226). Surely, however, Freud would have been confounded immediately by Mahler's erratic gait, which others described as a neurotic tic. "It wasn't possible to walk with him step-by-step, he always took three normal steps and then a short step, it was a nervous condition" (anonymous interviewee recorded in Mahler 1993). Nonetheless, the two walked and talked together, and they listened to each other deeply.

It helped. Mahler felt heard. On the train home Mahler composed a poem to his wife, Alma, that reads like a tribute to the success of Freud's therapeutic listening—"The tireless throb of torment ended. At last united in one single chord. My timid thoughts and my tempestuous feelings blended" (Pollock 1990, p.338). "It was only in the last year of life," Alma said, "when excesses of suffering had taught him the meaning of joy that his natural gaiety broke through the clouds" (A. Mahler 1973, p.120).

Engaging our grief

As Mahler turned his grief into music, I wonder about what we can do with our grief. Even years after significant losses in my own life, intense feelings of grief can come upon me so unexpectedly—while standing at the kitchen sink washing dishes, or at the gym in the midst of a workout. At other times, I know it is never far from me; grief has become a part of me. Where and when do you feel your grief? How do you deal with it? What does it compel you to do?

If you grieve "instrumentally," you prefer to do things constructively and keep busy with projects. Or, if you grieve "intuitively," you emote and share feelings more openly with others. According to gender stereotypes, men are more often instrumental grievers and women are intuitive grievers. However, that is not always the case. More typically, each one of us combines some elements of both styles of grieving in our own unique blended style of grief.

As grief psychotherapist Julia Samuel says, "we all need to find ways of expressing our grief, and it doesn't matter what the way is" (2018, p.239). Along with talking to family or friends, or writing a book or journal, some might find comfort in music, or in silence, in drawing or painting, or in talking to a therapist or counselor.

Confronted by loss, it is common to begin the grieving process by repeating the story to whomever is available to listen. Reflecting on the sudden death of her husband, Joan Didion said, "I must have repeated the details of what happened to everyone who came to the house in those first weeks" (2005, p.5).

I have no memory of telling anyone the details, but I must have done so, because everyone seemed to know them…the story they had was in each instance too accurate to have been passed from hand to hand. It had come from me. (p.5)

Nine months after her husband's death, Didion began to come to grips with her loss through writing. Her purpose in writing *The Year of Magical Thinking* was to try to make sense of the period of time following her loss:

> the weeks and then months that cut loose any fixed idea I had ever had about death, about illness, about probability and luck, about good fortune and bad, about marriage and children and memory, about grief, about the ways in which people do and do not deal with the fact that life ends, about the shallowness of sanity, about life itself. (p.7)

For others, grief prompts them to get up and move. They become more physically active. Exercising more, they might take up a sport, or train to run a half or full marathon for the first time, or take on even bigger challenges. Some trek the five hundred miles across northern Spain along the ancient pilgrimage route—the Camino de Santiago—to Santiago de Compostela (McManus 2014). Running a marathon or walking the Camino are ways to engage and express feelings by giving them physical shape, and spiritual meaning and purpose. One year after the death of her father, hospice chaplain Kerry Egan (2004) set out on the Camino to come to grips with her grief.

Both women and men undertake this kind of adventurous "transformative travel." It offers a form of therapy by presenting opportunities to break free of old habits and routines, to be resourceful and solve problems, to face our fears, to learn about ourselves, and to apply what we have learned to other aspects of our lives (Kottler 2010, pp.284–285).

There is something about the timing being right for this kind of spiritual journey. In the prologue to her book, *Steps out of Time: One Woman's Journey on the Camino*, American academic Katharine Soper said:

Faced with a milestone birthday, the death of my father, an empty nest, professional uncertainty, and for the first time in my life limitations imposed by health, I suddenly felt vulnerable—acutely mortal. Propelled by all of this...I decided to leave everything behind and head for Santiago de Compostela. (2013, p.iv)

Confronting midlife, English journalist Geoffrey Moorhouse went to the Sahara desert. "It was because I was afraid that I had decided to attempt a crossing of the great Sahara desert, from west to east, by myself and by camel," he said (1974, p.13).

I was a man who had lived with fear for nearly forty years... To live one's life in fear is something much less spectacular and much more commonplace in everyone's experience, I believe, than most of us are prepared to admit or even able to identify. (p.16)

Moorhouse travelled an incredible distance—about two thousand miles in all. He crossed Mauritania, passed through Timbuktu in Mali, and he made it as far as Tamanrasset, in southern Algeria, at which point he was forced to stop, less than halfway to his ultimate goal of reaching the Nile in Egypt. Before facing the journey home to England, Moorhouse rested at the hermitage of missionary Charles de Foucauld (1858–1916) in Assekrem, high up in the mountains about 60 miles north of Tamanrasset. "I had made a kind of peace with myself," he said (p.286). Sitting on the floor of Foucauld's small chapel with his back to the stone wall, he reflected: "This place was another reference point, to be used in times to come. It was one of many, and without them I would have been quite lost" (p.286).

As a young man, Norwegian explorer Erling Kagge went south. He skied alone across Antarctica all the way to the South Pole without radio contact in search of silence and of himself. "The quieter I became, the more I heard," he said (2017, p.14). He later went to the North Pole as well, and to the summit of Mount Everest. Now he searches for silence closer to home— in quiet moments before waking, in his daily commute, and in music, in the silences *between* notes, from dance music beat drops to Beethoven. "The silence I'm after," Kagge said, "is the silence within" (p.25).

I tend to think about silence as a practical method for uncovering answers to the intriguing puzzle that is yourself, and for helping to gain new perspective on whatever is hiding beyond the horizon (p.105)

Silence is about rediscovering, through pausing, the things that bring us joy... In knowing oneself, you know others. (p.85)

Kagge's sage advice for each of us is this—"You have to find your own South Pole" (p.128).

Maybe your South Pole is the Appalachian Trail, or going on a spiritual retreat. Or perhaps it is being by yourself in your car in solitude amidst traffic, in silence, or when a particular song comes on the radio and stirs your thoughts and feelings. Maybe it is paddling a kayak, or sitting quietly at your kitchen table, or in a favorite chair, calling forth special memories over a cup of coffee, or just taking a moment or two to listen to yourself breathe. Or it is standing in the shower, with a few precious moments to yourself before the demands of the world take over your day.

Your own South Pole might even be walking silently around an art gallery alone, giving yourself the time and space to stop and look deeply into a painting that catches your eye, and then allowing yourself to feel your feelings as they come to the surface. That is exactly what happened to writer Peter Schjeldahl (2016). At the Pace Gallery in New York City he attended an exhibition of paintings by American abstract artist Mark Rothko (1903–1970).

Rothko had said of his massive rectangular color panels, painted mostly in bold dark hues, that he was not interested "in relationships of form or color or anything else."

> I'm interested only in expressing basic human emotions—tragedy, ecstasy, doom, and so on—and the fact that lots of people break down and cry when confronted with my pictures shows that I *communicate* those basic human emotions. (Quoted in Rodman 1957, p.93)

Schjeldahl joked at first, "That's a lot to claim for fuzzy rectangles on paper or canvas" (2016, p.27). Yet he too admitted to feeling a "lyrical quality of heartbreak" while viewing one of Rothko's pictures, painted in 1955, with its dusky panels of lilac-gray, sea-blue, and a dominant black that, he said, seemed alternately, "to advance, as a clenched mass, and to recede, as infinite depth." Still, he said, "you might register it differently" (p.27).

Wherever you and your South Pole happen to be, the important thing is to be present to your feelings when they arise;

feeling and expressing emotions connect us more deeply to ourselves and to others.

In this chapter, we acknowledged the potential of our own transformative spiritual journey. We reviewed some ways to learn more about ourselves, by describing ourselves, exploring details of the stories we tell about ourselves—the stories that we are—and understanding the importance of being present to our feelings that demand expression. We raised questions to draw out our feelings about topics we might prefer to keep hidden from view because they are so painful, such as death and grief.

With Gustav Mahler as our guide, we learned that even amidst tremendous pain and suffering, there remains the potential for hope and joy. We heard from him how music was fundamental to his psychological and spiritual well-being. As Bruno Walter put it:

> Just as he expressed questions and yearning in music, so it was music, in turn, that kept questions and yearning alive within him and kindled them ever anew, for music has an irresistible power to guide the soul in the direction of the Beyond. (1941, pp.132–133)

Ultimately, Mahler experienced mystical healing through music, in the transfiguration from death into life. "Strange!" he said, "When I hear music—even while I conduct—I can hear quite definite answers to all of my questions and feel entirely clear and sure. Or rather, I feel quite clearly that they are no questions at all" (quoted in Walter 1941, p.153).

What I think Mahler appreciated through music is "optimal experience," or what psychologist Mihaly Csikszentmihalyi called "flow." As Csikszentmihalyi put it, people who describe "flow" experiences mention at least one, and often all, of the following:

> First, the experience usually occurs when we confront tasks we have a chance of completing. Second, we must be able to concentrate on what we are doing. Third and fourth, the concentration is usually possible because the task undertaken has clear goals and provides immediate feedback. Fifth, one acts with a deep but effortless involvement that removes awareness from the worries and frustrations of everyday life. Sixth, enjoyable experiences allow people to exercise a sense of control over their actions. Seventh, concern for the self disappears, yet paradoxically the sense of self emerges stronger after the flow experience is over. Finally, the sense of the duration of time is altered; hours pass by in minutes, and minutes can stretch out to seem like hours. The combination of all these elements cause a sense of deep enjoyment that is so rewarding people feel that expending a great deal of energy is worthwhile simply to be able to feel it. (2008, p.49)

Csikszentmihalyi documented how any activity can induce a sense of flow, such as the satisfying flow of thought, or work. It could be the joy of bodily movement in sport, exercise, dancing, sex, yoga, and the martial arts. Or it might be induced by reading, and sensory experiences of seeing, tasting, and listening, such as listening to music.

REFLECTION

Have you ever experienced "flow" in any of your favorite activities?

Chapter 6

FEELING HEARD AND UNDERSTOOD

It allowed me to settle—settle into myself.
Once I realized I was being heard, it allowed me to relax.
—Laura, hospice volunteer

In this chapter, we will consider who our listeners have been in our lives, and how we can learn more about listening to others by reflecting on our own experiences of feeling heard and understood. What does it feel like when someone really listens to you? This is a question I ask new volunteers in training sessions I teach about spirituality, grief and bereavement, about how listening helps, and how to become a better listener. And it is a question that I asked a small sample of hospice palliative care volunteers in a research study I completed recently.

The hospice palliative care volunteers I interviewed shared stories with me about times when they received listening from significant people in their lives. And they described how during these moments they felt settled and relaxed, confident, empowered, joyful, moved to tears, embraced, and loved. That is the positive power of listening that volunteers and other learners can draw upon from their own experience and offer to others.

Ten volunteers with a hospice in southeastern Ontario agreed to participate in my research study. They included seven women and three men, ranging in age from 24 to 81. Eight were retired from professional occupations, another was in a transitional phase of life between being employed and moving into retirement, and one was a university graduate student. Each expressed some sort of spiritual practice, from mindfulness meditation to yoga, to attending church services, or singing in church choirs. Their experience in hospice palliative care ranged from one year to more than 30 years.

Each volunteer provided informed and written consent to participate in an interview with me that lasted about an hour. During each interview, I was an "active listener" and helped each participant to tell her or his stories in her or his own way and own words.

First, I asked participants to describe themselves in a few words, and to share some details about their individual life histories, including significant relationships in their lives, their spirituality, and how they saw their roles as hospice palliative care volunteers. Next, I asked them to describe themselves as a listener, and what they felt constitutes good listening. Finally, I invited them to recall a particular time in their lives when they felt listened to by another person and received their full attention. Then I asked them to tell me a story about that experience. Their story about being listened to by another person, or the lack of listening they received, provided the central focus of the interview.

All the participants began by commenting on how they have the freedom of time and energy to devote to their roles as hospice palliative care volunteers. One volunteer said, "I have time and the energy, and volunteering seems like a compassionate way to spend some of that time and energy." Another volunteer talked about his freedom from financial worries at an older stage in life.

In comparison with his father, he commented that he is freer financially and emotionally than his father ever was. "Every day for me is worry-free," he said. "My father was never worry-free." He also reflected on the psychological freedom of being older now than his father was when he died. He described this freedom in terms of "uncharted territory."

One volunteer talked about being free to devote herself to what she believed is her true calling and vocation in life. "As a volunteer I'm doing what I want to do now," she said. "I see it as my life's work." All of the participants said that volunteering in hospice palliative care is for them an "honor," "privilege," and a "gift."

Each of the volunteers talked about the importance of listening in their roles in hospice palliative care. One said, "We all have different traits, but if you can't listen you can't be a palliative care volunteer." I will show you some of those different traits. They have to do with role models for listening, emotional needs, and styles of listening. In the excerpts below I use pseudonyms to protect their confidentiality.

Role models for listening

The kinds of role models for listening that the volunteers talked about included their parents, professional counselors, teachers, colleagues, and spouses. Sadly, one volunteer talked about the lack of listeners she has had in her life.

Parents

One volunteer talked about what she learned about listening from her mother. "My mother taught me that if I was listening I was going to learn a lot in life," she said, "and that stuck with me."

Robert: Did your mom listen to you?

Ellen: All the time.

Robert: What do you remember about the way she listened to you?

Ellen: My mother was a very busy woman. But when she came home from work, we would have our dinner, and she would sit and say, "How was your day?" And she meant it. You knew it was all she really cared about. That's how I knew my mother was listening. And she never forgot a thing. We knew that when mom got home she was going to give us her full and undivided attention. And we always felt listened to. My mom who's been gone for so long is with me every day.

Conversely, another volunteer talked about the lack of listening she received from her parents.

Robert: How did your parents listen to you growing up?

Laura: They didn't. Emotions were never talked about, and listening is not something that was ever modeled in our family.

Counselors

One volunteer talked about how she valued the support of her parents growing up, but when she needed someone to talk to when she was going through a "burnt-out phase, feeling anxious," she turned to a professional counselor, who she said was "gifted in listening."

Teachers

In the absence of parents as listeners and as role models for listening, some volunteers talked about receiving attentive listening for the first time in their lives as adults. These occurrences of listening didn't come in therapeutic relationships with counselors or psychotherapists. Rather, they happened spontaneously and unexpectedly with teachers and colleagues.

One volunteer described a turning point in her life when she was 30 years old and a student in law school. She recalled taking part in a role-play exercise about how to interview clients. In the role play she was interviewed by two different members of the law faculty. She described how the first interviewer (male) "talked a lot, gave a lot of information, and focused on legally relevant details." Then she described how the second interviewer (female) "just watched and waited until my answer was over, and then her questions arose from what was said, not from some other agenda."

Reflecting on this experience, she said:

I can still cry about it. Even though it was a role play, I really felt like someone was allowing me space. I felt listened to by my female colleague. It felt infinitely more powerful. I can remember it as if it were yesterday... When someone really asks you a question you have the opportunity to be reflective. It makes you wholly present, you are the center of somebody's focus. What a shame it took so long to receive in my life, it was a life-changing moment for me, and has stayed with me all my life.

Colleagues

Another volunteer received listening in mid-career from a colleague at work. Again, this was the first time this volunteer said he felt really listened to in his life. "My mother was not a good listener," he said, "and my father was absent... Good listening to me and good listening by me are both fairly recent things in my life."

He described how a conversation with his colleague during a training session about listening in their line of work turned into a kind of coaching session between them. This volunteer described how his listener paid full and close attention to him and helped him reassess his goals in life.

> I must've said something about how much space I wanted to take up in this world, to be bold and ambitious, or small and insignificant. And I remember her almost pleading with me to be bold. *And then she listened to me.* Before then I was in the wilderness not knowing what good listening was, and I was blessed with the good fortune to meet this person. That changed everything.

Robert: Do you remember what that felt like?

Allen: It felt huge, first of all, very warm, and intimate. It was a feeling of the heart. It hit me at the most intimate level. When a person is reaching out to you that way, there's a personal element focused on you that you can't help in that situation but feel a warmth, an intensity, love.

It was a blessing that I've carried with me. It was through that experience that I'm able to articulate today whether to be big or small.

You need somebody to listen to you, and you need to talk through that sort of thing in order to even realize that something like that might be an issue in your life. I had the good fortune to be introduced to that woman, and that changed everything for me.

Similarly, another volunteer described a time in her 40s during a vocational training session when she felt listened to attentively by another person. It was the first time she had ever felt really listened to, and she realized what she had been missing in her life until that point.

"Unlike talking with friends, it wasn't until I had that kind of experience that I finally understood what listening really was," she said, "and it shifted everything for me."

Robert: What did that kind of listening feel like to you?

Laura: A sadness that it wasn't there before. A grief that that was missing.

Robert: Can you take me into that experience? What made it so effective?

Laura: It allowed me to settle. Settle into myself. Once I realized I was being heard, it allowed me to relax. Then I was able to delve deeper into my thoughts. I felt embraced by the other person's whole being and that was so powerful. I felt completely understood, and loved.

Spouses

Another volunteer talked about the scarcity of good listeners in his life. Then he mentioned his wife, who he said is able to ask the "right kinds of questions."

Robert: What does it feel like to be asked the right questions?

Gary: Joy! You're uplifted because someone's not just listening but understanding. Also stillness. Somebody gives you confidence, because they are letting you experience what you are experiencing.

No listener role models

Sadly, another volunteer, in her 70s, said sincerely, "I've never really had anyone listen to me."

Emotional needs

Most of the volunteers expressed deep emotional needs extending from relationships in their families growing up. For example, three volunteers expressed longing for connections with emotionally distant or absent parents. One of them described herself from childhood as the designated family caregiver. She looked after the physical and emotional needs of other members of her family, including her single mom, a younger sister living with a disability, and other extended family members struggling with complex social issues, including alcoholism.

"For whatever reason," she explained, "when I was a little girl, I was the one who people went to for help and support." Later on, she became the primary caregiver for her mother when she was dying. Because of the caregiver role she had learned as a young child, she believed that volunteering in hospice care "comes naturally" to her.

From her caregiver role she also knew how important it was to address unfinished business, or what she called "un-dones" in life, for others and for herself.

Robert: What did you need? What did you long for as a child?

Ellen: A dad [tears].

Another volunteer described himself first as a "people person," and then as an "intimacy junkie," someone who "likes to help people" and who seeks emotional connections in relationships. He was the middle child in his family, raised in a household of "strong women," and with an emotionally distant father.

And another volunteer described herself as a "trier"— someone who has tried tirelessly throughout her life to heal estranged and broken relationships in her family, with little success.

Ann: As a volunteer, I'm driven by need.

Robert: What is that need?

Ann: No idea. Possibly to keep busy. I couldn't live my life without doing volunteer work. It makes me happy, and I haven't been happy most of my life. Also, there's the fear that someday I might need palliative care myself. If I give it, maybe I'll get it back. But I don't really believe that. I'd like to believe it. But I don't think I do. I don't think being good and nice gets you good and nice back. I don't think the world is like that anymore. I'm not that naïve anymore.

Robert: Do you feel like you deserve it?

Ann: I think everyone deserves it.

Robert: But what about *you*?

Ann: [Silence] I think the closest I've ever come to someone really caring for me is in being a hospice volunteer.

Another volunteer described a lonely childhood longing for her mother's attention and listening—a loneliness that persists into her late 50s, and is especially painful for her now amidst fading hope for things to be different in her relationship with her mother.

Laura: My parents are both 85 now and I think their capacity for listening is diminishing. About six months ago I said to my mom, "I'm feeling really sad."

Robert: What did she say?

Laura: She changed the subject.

Robert: How did that make you feel?

Laura: On the one hand it felt very familiar. Like, did I really expect anything different? I felt shut down, like she was saying, "Take it somewhere else to talk about that." And there's a great sadness that comes with that. She's not going to change now. [Silence] I've heard that people make some big changes when they're dying, they open up in all sorts of ways. So it's not that my mother will *never* change. There's always the possibility. But at this time, she doesn't want to go there. She likes to keep the façade that everybody's happy.

Styles of listening

For most of the volunteers I interviewed, role models for listening and enduring emotional needs formed and shaped their styles of listening to others in hospice palliative care.

Scanning for cues and making connections

One volunteer said, "I try to read what's going on in any situation, get a feel. I feel attuned to others." Another one described how in conversations he listens for cues or what he calls "nuggets" of information that might serve as openings to potentially deeper conversations. "From a little nugget," he said, "you can move into the *intimacy zone* with a topic of real importance." He described his style of listening as asking questions and probing a little bit to give others an opening for deeper conversations.

Being present

One volunteer said that "presence" is the most important thing to listen fully. She said:

> The last patient I was with who died was unresponsive. And as I sat with her holding her hand I felt like I was still listening to her. That connection was there. I was listening even though there were no words.

Slowing down

One volunteer talked about the kind of energy she brings to her role. "I'm different as a volunteer," she said.

It's completely different than in everyday life. I'm a busy person. But I slow down when I'm there. It's a completely different me. That's also the attraction for me. I get home and I feel good. I've accomplished something and for me it makes a difference. I just want to stay home and enjoy the feeling.

Being strong

"The last thing a dying person needs is someone terrified or blubbering at their side," one volunteer said. "I rise to fulfill the role." However, she admitted that it is easier to stay strong and calm for others who are not one's own family members. She described how she hopes to listen "profoundly" to others. "That kind of listening has become essential in my relationships," she said, "I am obliged and delighted to listen to others the same way."

As a listener, she described how she "adopted the technique" she learned in law school. Yet part of that technique involved categorizing and searching for answers. "I try not to do that now" she said, "I try to wait. I try not to find an answer unless I'm asked. It takes discipline and self-awareness." Now, she says, "I feel empowered to observe things in a different way." Mindful of the power of listening and of listeners who create and hold space for others, she described how listeners have power over others. She said:

Being in the room, being fully present and important, listeners have to be really careful not to deflate others by cutting them off. By opening up a conversation you have to be really careful about how to end it also. The best way to do it is to be honest and transparent, and by setting your own boundaries.

Listening from the heart

One volunteer talked about the emotional impact on her of being a listener for others. "People say things, and you carry them in your heart. It's here in my heart, and I remember them."

Another volunteer described listening from the heart as follows:

> You have to listen with your ears and with your heart too. It's like looking at the person with compassion. Gesture, touch, posture, showing interest are all important. It's about having your heart attuned to others with compassion and love that makes the connection.

Inviting people to tell stories

Another volunteer talked about how he appreciates the stories people tell, including his own, and how they provide a narrative identity, how he comes to know patients through the stories they tell. As a hospice volunteer, he talked about learning to be less of a storyteller and more of a story listener, with more tolerance and appreciation for silence.

In this chapter, we have explored how a small sample of hospice palliative care volunteers understand and appreciate the importance of listening in their lives and in their roles. They showed us how their styles of listening to others were influenced and shaped by their own deeply moving accounts of receiving, or longing to receive, good listening from others in their lives, including parents, professional counselors, teachers and colleagues, and spouses.

When author and educator Nancy Kline talked about her own experience of her mother's listening, she said:

My mother's listening was not ordinary. Her attention was so immensely dignifying, her expression so seamlessly encouraging, that you found yourself thinking clearly in her presence, suddenly understanding what before had been confusing, finding a brand-new, surprising idea. You found excitement where there had been tedium. You faced something. You solved a problem. You felt good again. … She simply gave attention. But the quality of that attention was catalytic. It would be forty years before I understood the power of what she was doing. (1999, p.15)

Receiving good listening may be especially pivotal in the lives of hospice palliative care volunteers, whose essential vocation it is to offer listening care to others.

As some volunteers were willing to share, their longing to feel heard and their motivations for listening stemmed from long-standing emotional needs. Since no family is perfect, many of us bear some hurts from the past. Unfortunately, in dysfunctional families there is the potential for chronic shame. As psychotherapist Patricia DeYoung put it:

If there's emotional trouble in the family, sensitive children try to manage it as best they can. They feel responsible for the well-being of fragile parents and vulnerable siblings. They spend their childhood offering emotional attunement beyond their years and doing without the emotional understanding they need. It's no wonder that some of them would one day make a career out of their attunement skills and their deep desire to see emotional hurts eased and relational brokenness repaired. (2015, p.78)

Emotional needs call for attention and support. First and foremost, we have to recognize and attend to our own needs and be aware of our motivations. I hope that the questions for self-reflection at the end of each chapter have helped you to slow down and be present to yourself as your own compassionate listener.

Yet hospice palliative care volunteers, as part of the healthcare team, also need support from volunteer managers, mentors, and peers. This raises questions about how best to teach active and empathic listening to volunteers, just as it is taught to professional healthcare staff in each of their disciplines, to ensure the safe and effective use of self.

The creative approaches to listening we reviewed in Chapter 2 suggest different ways that listening may be taught. These approaches included Dr. Rita Charon's method of "close reading" in her practice of narrative medicine, which she adapted from narrative theory (Charon 2017), listening being like a dance, in gesture and stillness; and Dr. Paul Haidet's use of jazz music as a metaphor to help medical students find and use their own authentic presence and "voice" as effective communicators (Haidet *et al.* 2017). And role play might take center stage, particularly for new volunteers for whom it might be a rare opportunity to observe how good listening is modeled, and even to receive it by having a skilled empathic listener listen to them with their full and undivided attention, perhaps for the very first time in their lives. Other methods include teaching a set of core principles about listening (Boudreau, Cassell, and Fuks 2009), and emphasizing attitude over technique (Martin *et al.* 2016).

This chapter suggests opportunities for more training for hospice palliative care volunteers in areas of reflective practice to enhance safe and effective use of self, including appropriate boundaries, and sensitivity to power imbalances and dynamics in healthcare environments. Moreover, it illuminates the need for volunteer managers to be mindful and sensitive to the emotional hurts and ongoing needs that volunteers bring to their roles in hospice palliative care, hurts and needs that are surely present to some degree in all healthcare workers in general.

By participating in the interviews presented in this chapter, the volunteers had an opportunity to receive active listening from me. Some of their reflections reveal, yet again, how rare and meaningful these kinds of conversations can be. Reflecting on his experience of the interview, one volunteer said:

> Some of the questions you asked made me probe myself, which is always interesting. I never have these types of conversations where people ask me questions that lead me to delve into my spiritual life or my fears. I'm actually getting a bit emotional just talking about it. I think about it often but I never talk about it because it's something that you don't usually talk about.

In the next, and final, chapter, I will tell you my story about feeling heard and understood, and what it means to me.

REFLECTION

- How did the listening you received from others in your life motivate and shape your own listening style?

- How did it affect your capacity for listening, and influence your approach to care in your role as a hospice palliative care volunteer?

- Have you experienced listening in ways that touched and moved your spirit?

CONCLUSION

Continuing the Journey

*Good listening to me and good listening by me
are both fairly recent things in my life.*

—Allen, hospice volunteer

Can I tell you a story from my life?

When I was a teenager, I escaped into movies. I was searching for something I could not articulate. One bright Saturday afternoon in Toronto I stepped into a repertory cinema and bought a ticket for a matinée of *My Dinner with Andre*. Two hours later I saw my life differently. Back in the sunlight, I knew then what I most needed to find—my listener.

My Dinner with Andre, written by and starring Andre Gregory and Wallace Shawn, was a unique film at the time in that no action takes place other than a conversation between the two characters in a fancy restaurant in Manhattan—Café des Artistes. It is an astonishing conversation between two old friends, two middle-aged men, both actors and playwrights.

Andre and Wally share stories about their experiences of work, the theater, their spouses, learning, ageing, and spirituality.

Andre tells some outlandish tales, and Wally listens skeptically, not quite sure what to believe. He is more practical than Andre. Still, he is an attentive, inquisitive, and appreciative listener. Wally too shares some of his stories, his thoughts, feelings, and questions about life and death, to which Andre provides thoughtful listening in return.

I was spellbound. I didn't know that conversations like that were possible. Andre and Wally revealed to me the magic of storytelling and listening relationships. And they showed me exactly what I was longing to receive from my dad.

Twenty years later I finally found my listener—three of them, in fact. I was in Milwaukee for an interview in the final phase of my application to become a certified member of the professional association I belonged to at the time, the National Association of Catholic Chaplains. Feeling nervous, I was prepared to talk about my professional skills as a chaplain, including how I believed that I could listen to others. What I did not expect was to receive the gift of listening myself.

I have had other people listen to me in my life, but the way these three interviewers listened to me stands out. They listened from the heart, with all of the qualities we have reviewed in this book. The kind of listening I received from them at that particular time was as radiant to me as the sunlight on that sidewalk outside the movie theater in Toronto. I knew then in my own experience as an adult the power of someone listening to me, understanding me, helping me understand myself, in a way that made me feel whole and complete, and very emotional.

Since then I have wondered if occurrences of receiving this kind of listening are just as rare and meaningful for other people too. In my talks for hospice palliative care volunteers on spirituality and grief, I have often asked participants about particular times that stand out for them of when they have felt heard and understood. That is what led me to interview the hospice palliative care volunteers in my research study, and to write this book.

My purpose in this book has been to try to connect our experiences of receiving listening with approaches to providing effective listening to others; to learn from our experiences of how others have listened to us in order to become better listeners ourselves.

"The heart finds relief in telling its troubles to another," St. Francis de Sales (1567–1622) said. "It is the best of remedies" (2002, pp.203–204, first published 1609). I wonder how he came to know that truth for himself. Who did he confide in? How did his listener or listeners touch his heart and inspire him in his own approach to caring for others?

Without knowing how he came to value listening so highly, we do know *how* he listened. According to a description provided by Francis's companion in ministry, St. Jane de Chantal (1572–1641):

> He received all comers with the same expression of quiet friendliness, and never turned anyone away, whatever his station in life; he always listened with unhurried calmness and for as long as people felt they needed to talk. He was so patient and attentive that you would have thought this was all he had to do. (Quoted in Stopp 1967, art. 46)

What is the source from which listeners drink that gives them life to enliven others? The answer will be different for each of us. But surely it will be in the form of a relationship with one or more significant persons in our lives.

In *The Other Way to Listen,* authors Byrd Baylor and Peter Parnall tell the story of a girl who learns from an old man about the value of silence, and what you can hear when you take the time to slow down and really pay attention to the world around you. As the story begins, the girl says, "I used to know an old man who could walk by any cornfield and hear the corn singing" (1997, p.1).

Walking together out into the desert, the girl and old man practice listening to the rocks, hills, and lizards. "Teach me," she urges the old man, "Just tell me how you learned to hear that corn."

He replies, "It takes a lot of practice. You can't be in a hurry." And she says, "I have the time" (p.1).

Eventually, the girl discovers the secret of "the other way to listen" in her joyous song to the hills. "All I know," she said, "is suddenly, I wasn't the only one singing."

> The hills were singing too. I stopped. I didn't move for maybe an hour. I never listened so hard in my life... It seemed to be the oldest sound in the world. (pp.23, 26)

This reminds me of a conversation I had once with a spiritual director at the end of a silent retreat a few years ago. She told me that when she was a young girl growing up on the prairie in Saskatchewan, her grandfather taught her how to listen to the sunset.

And it helps me appreciate that not all the silences I shared with my dad were painful ones.

One winter night when I was a very young child, my dad came home from work and took me for a skate on the river that went through our town. From one end to the other we skated in the dark, and in silence. The only sound between us was of our skates scraping the ice. In the summers I remember as a teenager how we sailed together on Lake Simcoe north of Toronto, mostly in silence, with only the sound of the breeze ruffling the sails. And I remember being with him as he died, with my sisters around his bed, late into the night, each of us attuned in silent vigil to the sound of his breathing, focused on being present to him physically, emotionally, and spiritually, listening to his cycles of different breathing sounds, until, finally, a deep resonant moan released his spirit. He died very gradually and peacefully, much like a leaf floating gently to the ground and then resting there. Still. Silent.

There have been many occasions in my life when I have had the opportunity to help others by listening to them. I have listened to my family, friends, colleagues, and my many patients over the years. I hope I listened well. But I know that there were many times when I didn't. Listening is a craft that requires constant attention and practice. There is always more to learn in each new experience.

We have reviewed how good listening leads us through cycles of picking up cues, and then responding with qualitative questions and other comments that invite additional details. How it requires checking perceptions and feelings, appreciating stillness and silence, and reflecting on connections to our own thoughts and feelings roused within us, our own stories. And how it requires close attention to the nuances of body language, such as making appropriate eye contact and monitoring the kind of energy we carry.

In the end, I think being a good listener comes down to being comfortable being yourself. But that is not as easy to accomplish as it might sound. It requires us to be *real* by knowing more about ourselves. It requires us to be *realistic* about our needs, abilities, and limitations, and about what listening can and cannot do. And it requires us to be ready to try to help others by daring to listen in the first place. Each of these aspects requires of us a generous spirit.

Going forward, there are at least three needs in hospice palliative care that I suggest call urgently for your listening skills as a volunteer, and mine as a chaplain.

The first need is what we have been talking about in this book: to help patients feel heard and understood. As Brian Nyatanga points out, "in palliative and end of life care the potential for misunderstanding or being misunderstood is real and therefore it is critical that our communication skills are the most advanced" (2017, p.360). A recent study focused specifically on this need. Researchers asked patients in palliative care, "Over the past two days, how much have you felt heard and understood by the doctors, nurses and hospital staff?" Their answers were recorded as "completely," "quite a bit," "moderately," "slightly," or "not at all," and they showed improvement when the question was repeated following an opportunity for the palliative care team to assess and treat each patient (Gramling *et al.* 2016, p.151).

Volunteers and chaplains were not uniquely identified among the "hospital staff" involved, but it is our special role to listen; it is what we do most prominently, and perhaps best. The listening we provide can help improve the quality of hospice palliative care.

The second need is to support staff. Hospice palliative care volunteers can help healthcare providers acknowledge grief in the workplace, and explore with them ways to express grief appropriately and effectively. Funk, Peters, and Roger (2017) illuminated this need in a recent qualitative study on the emotional labor of personal grief in palliative care. "Based on our research," Funk (2017) said, "I would recommend encouraging staff to recognize that expressing grief is normal and is OK—to de-stigmatize it in the workplace."

So many participants made comments that indicated that they felt it was unprofessional to show or even perhaps to feel grief when residents die. Some made very critical comments about others that were believed to be "too caring" or show too much distress when a patient dies. Just opening up these discussions gently with staff perhaps at times when they are not experiencing acute grief, could be helpful. (Funk 2017)

In this book, we have explored the very depths of grief and reflected on creative ways to express it and maybe even transform it into something beautiful. Gustav Mahler was our guide to deeper self-discovery. I hope you now feel better prepared to guide others.

The third need has to do with continuing to explore more about spirituality in our rapidly changing world, and what it means for us and especially for our patients and their loved ones in hospice palliative care who are facing the existential crisis of death approaching. Spirituality is woven into the very fabric of our being, in our living and in our dying, yet it is so difficult to define and articulate. It is a largely ineffable, mysterious quality of life (e.g. Manning 2012).

According to Puchalski *et al.*, spirituality is "the aspect of humanity that refers to the way individuals seek and express meaning and purpose, and the way they express their connectedness to the moment, to self, to others, to nature and the significant or sacred" (2009, p.887). It is an essential component of providing high-quality palliative care, and it requires listening.

Researchers John Cacioppo and William Patrick help us understand why a spirituality of listening is so important. In their book *Loneliness: Human Nature and the Need for Social Connection*, they point out the following trend:

In 1985, when researchers asked a cross-section of Americans, "How many confidants do you have?" the most common response to the question was three. In 2004, when researchers asked again, the most common response—made by twenty-five percent of the respondents—was none. One-quarter of these twenty-first-century Americans said they had no one at all with whom to talk openly and intimately. (2008, p.247)

You can imagine what the data would show today.

In our frenetic, chatty world of digital sound bites, tweets, and talking points, it seems that we have never been so immediately connected to so many people around the world, and yet all so superficially. I believe that taking the time to really listen is more important now than ever before, and it is likely one of the most generous and meaningful gifts we can offer to each other.

Reports from the Office for National Statistics suggest the UK has the highest rates of loneliness when compared with the rest of the European Union (Nyatanga 2017, p.360). As Nyatanga points out, "loneliness can result from being disadvantaged, discriminated upon, inequality, lack of control, lack of independence, lack of choice and options. Some of these factors are synonymous with feelings patients experience in end of life care" (p.360).

I believe that we long to tell our stories and risk sharing our feelings with others capable of listening so that we might not feel so alone and isolated in this world. By taking the time to listen we can help meet the desperate human need that I think we all feel at significant moments in our lives to connect with others spiritually at a deep level of understanding, and to feel heard.

What I have tried to demonstrate in this book is a spirituality of listening that offers a way for you to connect more deeply with the significant or the sacred dimension of life—in feelings of grief and joy, in music and in silence, and always through our relationships with others and with ourselves, in our stories. For me, listening has become a spiritual practice that shapes my way of living; it gives me meaning and purpose. And listening is a way of providing care that holds so much potential for helping and possibly even healing others and ourselves where we hurt the most.

Thank you for listening to me. By being present as a reader, you have helped me sort out some of my thoughts and feelings about myself as a listener, the sources from which I drink as a caregiver, my pain and my healing, and the role listening plays in our service to others near the end of life. I hope you have found in these pages something to help you on your own path towards becoming a better listener in the healing work you do as a hospice palliative care volunteer.

I have enjoyed having you with me on this journey.

Driving south from Burlington, Vermont, Interstate 89 arcs eastward to Montpelier. It is here, along this stretch of highway, where I drove with my dad. And it is here, in my imagination, where I pick up my son and continue the journey.

Breaking the silence between us as we drive together, my son asks, "Can I tell you something?"

I have been preparing for this moment his whole life.

"Of course," I answer, "that's why I'm here."

AFTERWORD

Being a hospice palliative care volunteer for over two decades, I fully understand the importance of good listening skills. I think you will agree that this book is invaluable to anyone who needs to communicate with someone who is at the end of life; a time when communicating becomes very difficult, sensitive, cautious, and fearful.

I cultivated most of my listening skills during my first seven years of volunteering, serving nearly a thousand people who came to finish their life's journey in a lovely old Victorian home, fondly known as the Guest House at the Zen Hospice Project, in San Francisco.

Zen Hospice had an excellent training program and I felt reasonably well prepared to embark on my journey of serving people who were dying in whatever way I could. When I began in 1996 at the Guest House, we had a plethora of ways to compassionately serve outside of the traditional ways volunteers typically serve in today's more restricted healthcare environment such as sitting at the bedside—sometimes overnight—bathing, cooking, feeding, washing clothes, foot massages, etc.

Guest House volunteers learned some good approaches to listening during one two-hour training session, which included some role-playing. As I began to serve our residents, I quickly discovered that being a good listener was going to take some time and more practice after one of the first residents I was visiting looked over and very politely asked, 'Could you please stop talking?'

As I looked back on that experience while reading Robert Mundle's book, I wished I had had it available to augment my initial training. His book reflects a depth of knowledge about listening that only comes through many years of experience at the bedside. Robert took me on a journey of reflection and rediscovery as he explained the variety of techniques I had to learn instinctively over many years.

Good listening is a learned skill. My teacher, Frank Ostaseski—founder of the Zen Hospice—taught me that to be a good intuitive listener you should be listening with 50 percent of your attention on the person speaking while keeping the other 50 percent on your own body and personal awareness. This approach helps to keep you connected as you bear witness to the dying person's journey.

The primary challenges for the volunteer in bearing witness to the journey are twofold. First, the individual who is dying may have been on their journey for perhaps years by the time they reach hospice. They have likely told their story too many times to too many people. They can be weary. Second, the volunteer has virtually no knowledge of that journey when beginning their part of this journey.

As a result, it typically takes several weekly visits for the volunteer to begin to establish sufficient trust that will nudge the dying person into going deeper in conversation, revealing where they really are on their journey—the first step in creating a connection that fosters compassion. The book *How Can I Help?* by Ram Dass and Paul Gorman beautifully describes what happens when the two find this place:

When our models of who we are fall away, we are free simply to meet and be together. And when this sense of being encompasses all—one another, the park, the rain, everything—separateness dissolves and we are united in compassion. (2003, p.38)

Robert has brought forth a spiritual roadmap that guides the volunteer on how to find that place where meaningful dialogue can begin. He presents methods and approaches that provide useful guidance as we encounter the uncertainties that surely will show themselves as the journey progresses, sometimes with grace, other times with suffering.

Another passage from *How Can I Help?* reflects on listening with an "intuitive mind" when the volunteer is faced with uncertainty while trying to be fully present to bear witness:

[T]his kind of listening to the intuitive mind is a kind of surrender based on trust. It's playing it by ear, listening for the voice within. ... As we learn to listen with a quiet mind, there is so much we hear. ... In other people we hear what help they really require, what license they are actually giving us to help, what potential there is for change. We can hear their strengths and their pain. We hear what support is available, obstacles must be reckoned with. (pp.111–112)

Listening is an art. Robert Mundle's book quite eloquently shows us why this is so. One must be a nimble listener, yet one who can be creative as well. The tools to help you achieve these abilities are here in this book.

On behalf of all the current and future hospice palliative care volunteers in the world, thank you, Robert, for this most useful contribution to help us better serve those who are dying and their families.

Greg Schneider

Founder and President, Hospice Volunteer Association

Founding Director and CEO, Hospice Educators

Affirming Life (HEAL) Project

REFERENCES

Adamle, K. and Ludwick, R. (2005) "Humor in hospice care: Who, where, and how much?" *American Journal of Hospice and Palliative Medicine 22*, 4, 287–290.

Arrupe, P. (2009) "Fall in Love." In *Finding God in All Things: A Marquette Prayer Book*. Milwaukee, WI: Marquette University Press.

Bailey, E.T. (2010) *The Sound of a Wild Snail Eating*. Chapel Hill, NC: Algonquin Books of Chapel Hill.

Bauby, J.D. (1997) *The Diving Bell and the Butterfly*. London: Fourth Estate.

Baylor, B. and Parnall, P. (1997) *The Other Way to Listen*. New York: Aladdin Paperbacks.

Boff, L. (1987) *Sacraments of Life, Life of the Sacraments: Story Theology*. Translated by John Drury. Washington, DC: Pastoral Press.

Boisen, A. (1936) *The Exploration of the Inner World: A Study of Mental Disorder and Religious Experience*. New York: Harper & Brothers.

Boston, P. and Mount, B. (2006) "The caregiver's perspective on existential and spiritual distress in palliative care." *Journal of Pain and Symptom Management 32*, 1, 13–26.

Boudreau, J.D., Cassell, E., and Fuks, A. (2009) "Preparing medical students to become attentive listeners." *Medical Teacher 31*, 22–29.

Brighton, L., Koffman, J., Robinson, V., Khan, S. *et al.* (2017) "'End of life could be on any ward really': A qualitative study of hospital volunteers' end-of-life care training needs and learning preferences." *Palliative Medicine 31*, 9, 842–852.

Brown, P., Alaszewski, A., Swift, T., and Nordin, A. (2011) "Actions speak louder than words: The embodiment of trust by healthcare professionals in gynae-oncology." *Sociology of Health and Illness 33*, 2, 280–295.

Buckman, R. (1988) *I Don't Know What to Say: How to Help and Support Someone Who Is Dying*. Toronto: Key Porter Books.

Burley-Allen, M. (1995) *Listening: The Forgotten Skill* (2nd edition). New York: John Wiley and Sons.

Butler, R. (2007) "Life Review." In J.E. Birren (ed.) *Encyclopedia of Gerontology: Age, Aging and the Aged*, Vol. 1 (2nd edition). San Diego, CA: Academic Press.

Cacioppo, J.T. and Patrick, W. (2008) *Loneliness: Human Nature and the Need for Social Connection*. New York: W.W. Norton & Company.

Carel, H. (2008) *Illness: The Cry of the Flesh*. Stocksfield: Acumen.

Chang, L. (2006) *Wisdom for the Soul: Five Millenia of Prescriptions for Spiritual Healing*. Washington, DC: Gnosophia Publishers.

Charon, R. (2005) "Narrative medicine: Attention, representation, affiliation." *Narrative 13, 3*, 261–270.

Charon, R. (2017) "Close Reading: The Signature Method of Narrative Medicine." In R. Charon, S. DasGupta, N. Hermann, C. Irvine, *et al. The Principles and Practice of Narrative Medicine*. New York: Oxford University Press.

Clary, P. (2010) "Poetry and healing at the end of life." *Journal of Pain and Symptom Management 40, 5*, 796–800.

Claxton-Oldfield, S. and Bhatt, A. (2017) "Is there a place for humor in hospice palliative care? Volunteers say 'Yes'!" *American Journal of Hospice Palliative Medicine 34, 5*, 417–422.

Claxton-Oldfield, S. and Jones, R. (2013) "Holding on to what you have got: Keeping hospice palliative care volunteers volunteering." *American Journal of Hospice and Palliative Care 30, 5*, 467–472.

Cohen, L. (1993) *Stranger Music: Selected Poems and Songs*. Toronto: McClelland and Stewart.

Coleridge, S.T. (1997) "Rime of the Ancient Mariner." In *Coleridge: The Complete Poems*. London: Penguin Books. (Original work published 1884.)

Cooper-White, P. (2004) *Shared Wisdom: Use of the Self in Pastoral Care and Counseling*. Minneapolis, MN: Fortress Press.

Cooper-White, P. (2007) *Many Voices: Pastoral Psychotherapy in Relational and Theological Perspective*. Minneapolis, MN: Fortress Press.

Csikszentmihalyi, M. (2008). *Flow: The Psychology of Optimal Experience*. New York: Harper Perennial Modern Classics. (Original work published 1990.)

Davies, R. (1994) *The Cunning Man: A Novel*. Toronto: McClelland and Stewart.

DeYoung, P.A. (2015) *Understanding and Treating Chronic Shame: A Relational/ Neurobiological Approach*. New York and London: Routledge.

Didion, J. (2005) *The Year of Magical Thinking*. New York: Vintage.

Drews, M.F. (2017) "The evolution of hope in patients with terminal illness." *Nursing 47*, 1, 13–14.

Dunphy, J. (2011) *Communication in Palliative Care: Clear, Practical Advice, Based on a Series of Real Case Studies*. London and New York: Radcliffe.

Egan, K. (2004) *Fumbling: A Pilgrimage Tale of Love, Grief and Spiritual Renewal on the Camino de Santiago*. New York: Random House.

Egan, K. (2016) *On Living*. London: Penguin.

eHospiceUSA (2016) "Statistics on volunteering and hospice." Accessed on 02/01/18 at www.ehospice.com/usa/Default/tabid/10708/ArticleId/ 18969.

Feder, S. (2004) *Gustav Mahler: A Life in Crisis*. New Haven, CT, and London: Yale University Press.

Floros, C. (2000) *Gustav Mahler: The Symphonies*. Translated from the German by Vernon and Jutta Wicker. Pompton Plains, NJ: Amadeus Press.

Francis, de Sales, Saint. (2002) *Introduction to the Devout Life*. New York: Vintage Books. (Original work published 1609.)

Frank. A.W. (2004) *The Renewal of Generosity: Illness, Medicine, and How to Live*. Chicago, IL, and London: University of Chicago Press.

Frank. A.W. (2005) "Generosity, Care, and a Narrative Interest in Pain." In D. Carr, J. Loeser, and D. Morris (eds) *Narrative, Pain, and Suffering*. Vol. 34 in *Pain, Research and Management*. Seattle, WA: IASP Press.

Frank, A.W. (2010) *Letting Stories Breathe: A Socio-Narratology*. Chicago, IL: University of Chicago Press.

Frank, A.W. (2013) The *Wounded Storyteller: Body, Illness, and Ethics* (2nd edition). Chicago, IL: University of Chicago Press.

Frank, A.W. (2017) "An illness of one's own: Memoir as art form and research as witness." *Cogent Arts and Humanities 4*, 1, 1343654. Accessed on 02/01/2018 at www.cogentoa.com/article/10.1080/23311983.2017.1343654.

Funk, L. (2017) Unpublished personal correspondence with Robert Mundle.

Funk, L., Peters, S., and Roger, K. (2017) "The emotional labor of personal grief in palliative care: Balancing caring and professional identities." *Qualitative Health Research 27*, 14, 2211–2221.

Gergen, K.J. (2009) *Relational Being: Beyond Self and Community*. New York and Oxford: Oxford University Press.

Gopnik, B. (2009) "'Golden Seams: The Japanese art of mending ceramics' at Freer." *The Washington Post*, March 3, 2009. Accessed on 02/01/2018 at www.washingtonpost.com/wp-dyn/content/article/2009/03/02/AR2009030202723.html.

Gramling, R., Stanek, S., Ladwig, S., Gajary-Coots, E., *et al.* (2016) "Feeling heard and understood: A patient-reported quality measure for the inpatient palliative care setting." *Journal of Pain and Symptom Management* 51, 2, 150–154.

Haidet, P., Jaracke, J., Yang, C., Teal, C., Street Jr., R., and Stuckey, H. (2017) "Using jazz as a metaphor to teach improvisational communication skills." *Healthcare 5*, 3, 41.

Haitink, B. (1996) *In Conducting Mahler*. Documentary film directed by Frank Scheffer. Allegri Films.

Halpern, J. (2001) *From Detached Concern to Empathy: Humanizing Medical Practice*. New York: Oxford University Press.

Hentoff, N. (2001) "Jazz: Beyond Time and Nations." In *The Nat Hentoff Reader*. Boston, MA: Da Capo Press.

Hitchens, C. (2017) "Hitchens on Literature." In *Christopher Hitchens: The Last Interview*. Brooklyn, NY, and London: Melvin House Publishing. First published in *Stop Smiling*, 20, April 2005.

HospiceUK. (2017) "Volunteering." Accessed on 02/01/18 at www.hospiceuk.org/about-hospice-care/volunteering-in-hospice-care.

James, H. (1984) "The Art of Fiction." In *Partial Portraits*. London: Macmillan and Company. (Original work published 1888.)

Kagge, E. (2017) *Silence in the Age of Noise*. Translated from the Norwegian by Beckie L. Crook. New York: Pantheon Books.

Kalanithi, P. (2016) *When Breath Becomes Air*. New York: Random House.

Kandula, N. (2013) "The power of listening to our patients." American Medical Association. Accessed on 02/01/2018 at www.youtube.com/watch?v=ISUqR7q0dk8.

Kellehear, A., Pugh, E., and Atter, L. (2009) "A home away from home? A case study of bedside objects in a hospice." *International Journal of Palliative Nursing 15*, 3, 148–152.

Kelley, M.M. (2010) *Grief: Contemporary Theory and the Practice of Ministry*. Minneapolis, MN: Fortress Press.

Kenyon, G.M. and Randall, W.L. (1997) *Restorying Our Lives: Personal Growth Through Autobiographical Reflection*. Westport, CT, and London: Praeger.

Klemperer, O. (1961) *Mahler Symphony No. 4*. London: EMI.

Kline, N. (1999) *Time to Think: Listening to Ignite the Human Mind*. London: Cassell.

Kottler, J.A. (2010) *On Being a Therapist* (4th edition). San Francisco, CA: Jossey-Bass.

Kübler-Ross, E. and Kessler, D. (2005) *On Grief and Grieving: Finding the Meaning of Grief through the Five Stages of Loss*. New York: Scribner.

Kurtz, E. and Ketcham, K. (1992) The *Spirituality of Imperfection: Storytelling and the Search for Meaning*. New York: Bantam.

MacDonald, K. (2009) "Patient-clinician eye contact: Social neuroscience and the art of clinical engagement." *Postgraduate Medicine 121*, 4, 1–9.

MacFarquhar, L. (2016) "A tender hand in the presence of death." *The New Yorker*, July 11 & 18. Accessed 02/01/2018 at www.newyorker.com/magazine/2016/07/11/the-work-of-a-hospice-nurse.

Mackenzie, C. (2006) "Imagining other lives." *Philosophical Papers 35*, 293–325.

Mackinlay, E. (2012) *Palliative Care, Ageing and Spirituality: A Guide for Older People, Carers and Families*. London: Jessica Kingsley Publishers.

Mahler, A. (1973) *Gustav Mahler: Memories and Letters*. D. Mitchell (ed.) (3rd edition). London: John Murray. (Original work published 1946.)

Mahler, G. (1966) *Symphony No. 4, G Major*. London: Ernst Eulenburg.

Mahler, G. (1993) "Remembering Mahler." *Mahler Plays Mahler: The Welte-Mignon Piano Rolls*. New York: Kaplan Foundation.

Manning, L. (2012) "Articulating the ineffable: Explorations into the spiritual lives of old women." *Journal of Religion Spirituality and Aging 24*, 3, 179–201.

Marcel, G. (2011) "On the Ontological Mystery." In B. Sweetman (ed.) *A Gabriel Marcel Reader*. South Bend, IN: St. Augustine's Press. (Original work published 1944.)

Martin, O., Rockenbauch, K., Kleinert, E., and Stöbel-Richter, Y. (2016) ["Effectively communicate active listening: Comparison of two concepts."] *Der Nervenarzt 88*, 9, 1026–1035. (Article in German.)

McBratney, S. (1994) *Guess How Much I Love You*. Somerville, MA: Candlewick Press.

McMahon, E.M. and Campbell, P.A. (1969) *Please Touch*. New York: Sheed and Ward.

McManus, B. (2014) *Redemption Road: Grieving on the Camino*. Dublin: Orpen Press.

Menninger, K. (1942) *Love Against Hate*. New York: Harcourt, Brace and Company.

Mills, M., Speck, P., and Coleman, P. (2011) "Listening and Enabling the Sharing of Beliefs and Values in Later Life." In P. Coleman (ed.) *Belief and Ageing: Spiritual Pathways in Later Life*. Bristol, UK: The Policy Press.

Moorhouse, G. (1974) *The Fearful Void*. New York: Clarkson N. Potter, Inc. Publishers.

Mowat, H., Bunniss, S., Snowden, A., and Wright, L. (2013) "Listening as health care." *Scottish Journal of Healthcare Chaplaincy 16*, 35–41.

Mundle, R. (2014) "Strong men don't cry, but I'm not strong anymore." *Illness, Crisis and Loss 22*, 4, 285–292.

Mundle, R. and Smith, B. (2013) "Hospital chaplains and embodied listening: Engaging with stories and the body in healthcare environments." *Illness, Crisis and Loss 21*, 2, 95–108.

Nouwen, H. (1972) *The Wounded Healer: Ministry in Contemporary Society*. New York: Doubleday.

Nouwen, H. (1976) *Reaching Out: The Three Movements of the Spiritual Life*. London: Collins.

Nyatanga, B. (2017) "Being lonely and isolated: Challenges for palliative care." *British Journal of Community Nursing 22*, 7, 360.

O'Brien, S. and Wallace, E. (2009) "Volunteers Working in a Tertiary Referral Teaching Hospital." In R. Scott and S. Howlett (eds) *Volunteers in Hospice and Palliative Care: A Resource for Voluntary Services Managers* (2nd edition). Oxford and New York: Oxford University Press.

Ofri, D. (2017) *What Patients Say, What Doctors Hear*. Boston, MA: Beacon Press.

Petty, T. (1994) "You Don't Know How It Feels." *Wildflowers*. Warner/Chappell Music.

Pollock, G. (1990) "Mourning Through Music: Gustav Mahler." In S. Feder, R.L. Karmel, and G.H. Pollock (eds) Psychoanalytic Explorations in Music. Madison, CT: International Universities Press.

Puchalski, C.M., Ferrell, B., Virani, R., Otis-Green, S., *et al.* (2009) "Improving the quality of spiritual care as a dimension of palliative care: The report of the consensus conference." *Journal of Palliative Medicine 12*, 10, 885–904.

Ram Dass and Gorman, P. (2003) *How Can I Help? Stories and Reflections on Service*. New York: Knopf.

Randall, W. (2012) "Beyond Healthy Aging: The Practice of Narrative Care in Gerontology." In L. English (ed.) *Adult Education and Health*. Toronto, Buffalo, and London: University of Toronto Press.

Randall, W.L. and McKim, A.E. (2008) *Reading Our Lives: The Poetics of Growing Old*. New York: Oxford University Press.

Randall, W., Prior, S., and Skarborn, M. (2006) "How listeners shape what tellers tell: Patterns of interaction in life-story interviews and their impact on reminiscence on elderly interviewees." *Journal of Aging Studies* 20, 4, 381–396.

Reik, T. (1983) *The Haunting Melody: Psychoanalytic Experiences in Life and Music.* New York: Da Capo Press.

Rodman, S. (1957) *Conversations with Artists.* New York: Devin-Adair Publishing Company.

Rubinstein, R.L. (1987) "The significance of personal objects to older people." *Journal of Aging Studies* 1, 3, 225–238.

Rumi. (1996) *The Essential Rumi.* Translated by Coleman Barks. New York: HarperCollins.

Sacks, O. (2007) "Lamentations: Music, Madness, and Melancholia." In *Musicophilia: Tales of Music and the Brain.* Toronto: Vintage Canada.

Samuel, J. (2018) *Grief Works: Stories of Life, Death, and Surviving.* Toronto: Doubleday Canada.

Sandoval, J. (2017) "Translator's Afterword." In J. Sandoval (ed.) *From the Monastery to the World: The Letters of Thomas Merton and Ernesto Cardenal.* Berkeley, CA: Counterpoint.

Saunders, C. (2006) "Foreword." (*Oxford Textbook of Palliative Medicine*, 3rd edition, 2004). In *Cicely Saunders: Selected Writings: 1958–2004.* New York: Oxford University Press.

Savage, J. (1996) *Listening and Caring Skills: A Guide for Groups and Leaders.* Nashville, TN: Abingdon Press.

Schjeldahl, P. (2016) "The dark final years of Mark Rothko." *The New Yorker*, December 19 & 26, 27. Accessed on 02/01/18 at www.newyorker.com/magazine/2016/12/19/the-dark-final-years-of-mark-rothko.

Scott-Maxwell, F. (1968) *The Measure of My Days.* London: Penguin.

Smith, D.H. (2005) *Partnership with the Dying: Where Medicine and Ministry Should Meet.* Lanham, MD: Rowman and Littlefield.

Soper, K. (2013) *Steps out of Time: One Woman's Journey on the Camino.* Ann Arbor, MI: Stellaire Press.

Stanworth, R. (2004) *Recognizing Spiritual Needs in People Who Are Dying.* New York: Oxford University Press.

Steiner, G. (1989) *Real Presences: Is There Anything in What We Say?* London and Boston, MA: Faber and Faber.

Stopp, E. (1967) *St. Francis de Sales: A Testimony by St. Chantal.* London: Faber and Faber.

Stroebe, M. and Schut, H. (1999) "The dual process model of coping with bereavement: Rationale and description." *Death Studies* 23, 3, 197–224.

Swayden, K.J., Anderson, K.K., Connelly, L.M., Moran, J.S., McMahon, J.K., and Arnold, P.M. (2012) "Effect of sitting vs. standing on perception of provider time at bedside: A pilot study." *Patient Education and Counseling* 86, 2, 166–171.

Sweet, V. (2017) *Slow Medicine: The Way to Healing.* New York: Riverhead Books.

Tapscott, S. (ed.) (1996) *Twentieth-Century Latin American Poetry: A Bilingual Anthology.* Austin, TX: University of Texas Press.

Taylor, J. (2008) *My Stroke of Insight: A Brain Scientist's Personal Journey.* New York: Viking.

Tibi-Lévy, Y. and Bungener, M. (2017) "Volunteering in Palliative Care in France: 'A Tough Job': Patient, Family, Caregiver, and Volunteer Perspectives." In J. Guajardo-Rosas (ed.) *Highlights on Several Underestimated Topics in Palliative Care.* InTech. Accessed on 02/01/2018 at www.intechopen.com/books/highlights-on-several-underestimated-topics-in-palliative-care/volunteering-in-palliative-care-in-france-a-tough-job-patient-family-caregiver-and-volunteer-perspec

Ueland, B. (1941) "Tell me more." *Ladies' Home Journal.* Philadelphia, PA: Curtis Publishing Company. Reprinted in B. Ueland (1993), *Strength to Your Sword Arm: Selected Writings.* Duluth, MN: Holy Cow! Press.

Vanier, J. (2007) *Our Life Together: A Memoir in Letters.* Toronto: HarperCollins Publishers.

Walter, B. (1941) *Gustav Mahler.* New York: Greystone Press.

Webb, C. (2016) *How to Have a Good Day: Harness the Power of Behavioral Science to Transform Your Working Life.* New York: Crown Business.

West, C. (2008) Interview. *Examined Life.* Documentary film by Astra Taylor. Zeitgeist Films.

Wheatley, M. (2002) *Turning to One Another: Simple Conversations to Restore Hope to the Future.* San Francisco, CA: Berrett-Koehler Publishers.

Wolterstorff, N. (1987) *Lament for a Son.* Grand Rapids, MI: William B. Eerdmans Publishing Company.

Worthington, D.L. (2008) "Communication skills training in a hospice volunteer training program." *Journal of Social Work in End-of-Life and Palliative Care* 4, 1, 17–37.

Znaimer, M. (1990) "Jean Vanier: A portrait in the first person." *The Originals,* Episode 24. Mississauga: Marlin Motion Pictures.

SUBJECT INDEX

AUTHOR INDEX

ABOUT THE AUTHOR

Robert Mundle is a registered psychotherapist and spiritual health practitioner who has spent the last 15 years working with patients and their loved ones in palliative care. He is a graduate of Yale Divinity School and the University of Toronto with degrees in music and theology. He completed a residency in specialized training for chaplains at the Hospital of St. Raphael, which is now part of Yale–New Haven Hospital in New Haven, Connecticut.

Robert currently lives in Kingston, Ontario, with his wife, Mi-Sook, and son, Christopher. When not at the hockey rink cheering as a hockey dad, he enjoys reading and collecting books, cooking Korean food, listening to Mahler, and playing the classical guitar.

How to Be an Even Better Listener is his first book.

Visit Robert's blog at www.robertmundle.com.